22 EB 1/3/83.

Anesthetic Exposure in the Workplace

Ellis N. Cohen, M.D.
Professor of Anesthesia
Stanford University

PSG Publishing Company, Inc.
Littleton, Massachusetts

Library of Congress Cataloging in Publication Data

Cohen, Ellis N
   Anesthetic exposure in the workplace.

   Includes bibliographical references and index.
   1.   Operating room personnel—Diseases and hygiene.
2.   Anesthetics—Toxicology.   3.   Anesthetics—Safety
measures.   4.   Dental personnel—Diseases and hygiene.
I.   Title.   [DNLM: 1.   Anesthetics—Adverse effects.
2.   Environmental exposure.   3.   Occupational medicine.
QV81 C678a]
RD32.3.C63   617'.96'028   79-16694
ISBN 0-88416-252-4

Printed in the United States of America.

International Standard Book Number: 0-88416-252-4

Library of Congress Catalog Card Number: 79-16694

To Sylvia

Partial support for these studies has been provided under Department of Health, Education and Welfare Grants OH 00622, OH 00775, Contract HSM 99-73-3, and Contract CDC 210-75-0007.

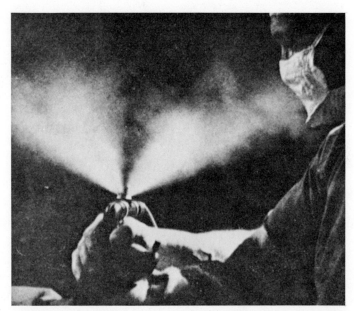

Anesthetic exit flow patterns from a Heidbrink valve revealed by smoke. (From Smith, W.D.A. et al. *Int Anesthesiol Clin.* 16:131–173, 1978. Reprinted by permission of the publisher, Little, Brown and Co., and of the author.)

CONTRIBUTORS

Charles L. Geraci, Jr., Ph.D.
Division of Physical Sciences and Engineering
National Institute for Occupational Safety and Health

Gale A. Mondry, J.D.
Associate Counsel for Medical Affairs
Stanford University

Charles E. Whitcher, M.D.
Professor of Clinical Anesthesia
Stanford University

CONTENTS

7 Role of Government 149
Charles L. Geraci, Jr.

8 Medical-Legal Implications 163
Gale A. Mondry

Remedies against Third Parties
Conclusions

INTRODUCTION

The past decade has witnessed growing concern regarding significant health problems associated with work in the operating room and dental operatory. It is estimated that in the United States alone, in excess of 214,000 physicians, nurses, technicians, dentists, and chairside assistants are occupationally at risk each year. Although these health hazards have been suggested to include increased spontaneous abortion, congenital anomalies, liver disease, female cancer, and decreased mental performance, firm evidence associating their etiology with the waste anesthetic gases remains to be established. Unfortunately, the animal data are inconsistent, and species variations have prevented development of an adequate experimental model. Nonetheless, some 20 epidemiologic surveys conducted in the United States and abroad confirm the presence of an occupational hazard, and a recent large-scale dental survey offers strong evidence for a positive cause-and-effect association with anesthetic gases.

The presence of an occupational hazard involving such large numbers of health professionals has not gone unnoticed. The National Institute for Occupational Safety and Health (NIOSH), after carefully reviewing all available animal and clinical data, has prepared a Criteria Document which defines the extent of the problem and suggests appropriate measures for its control. Included in this document are specific recommendations for limits of waste anesthetic gases in the workplace, means for notification of exposed individuals of their work-associated risk, descriptions of various measuring devices capable of monitoring concentrations of waste anesthetic gas, and specific methods for evacuating these gases from the breathing atmosphere.

The present volume attempts to bring these many considerations into appropriate focus. Chapter 1 presents a brief historical overview. Chapter 2 defines precise concentrations of waste anesthetic gases present in the operating room and dental operatory under a variety of clinical conditions. The next two chapters provide relevant background information culled from a wide base of experimental laboratory and human epidemiologic studies which serve to establish the extent of the health hazard. The data are emphasized by discussions in Chapter 5 suggesting mechanisms of toxicity associated with exposure to the trace anesthetic gases. These presentations are in turn followed by a detailed description of methods for monitoring the waste anesthetic gases and means of removing them from the atmosphere. Chapter 7 discusses the role of government in the education, prevention, and control of health hazards present in the workplace. The final chapter is concerned with legal considerations, including possible implications of failure to protect and inform the worker by the responsible employer(s).

These discussions provide adequate data to enable each reader to come to an independently based conclusion as to the seriousness of the health risk(s) involved. In reaching such a conclusion, cost-to-benefit ratios must be considered, as well as potential legal implications attendant to noncompliance. Those individuals positively influenced by the data will find useful the in-detail description of specific protective measures that may be taken to monitor and reduce exposure to the waste anesthetic gases. Individuals who remain unconvinced will at least have had the opportunity to review the available information and arrive at a knowledgeable decision.

1 Historical Perspectives

At age 22, Sir Humphrey Davy (1800) published his remarkable experiments with "dephylogisticated nitrous air." In these pioneering studies, Davy not only convincingly demonstrated the fallacy of the then accepted theory that dephylogisticated nitrous air was the source of contagious disease, but also offered the first written suggestion that this gas possessed useful anesthetic properties. Having observed a stupifying response in several animal species following their inhalation of nitrous air, Davy conducted a series of self-experiments which, on at least one occasion, consisted of personal use of the gas for pain alleviation.

> ...I experienced an extensive inflammation of the gum, accompanied with great pain, which equally destroyed the power of repose and of consistent action. On the day when the inflammation was most troublesome, I breathed three large doses of nitrous oxide. The pain diminished after the first four or five respirations...

This self-application of nitrous oxide by Davy probably represents its first recorded use for anesthetic purpose in humans.

It remained for an American dentist, Horace Wells (1847), to apply this significant discovery to the clinical setting by allowing his student, John Riggs, to administer nitrous oxide to Wells himself for extraction of a diseased molar. Although Wells' painless surgical extraction quickly served to establish nitrous oxide as a successful dental analgetic, extended use of the gas in general surgery was slow in coming. There were several important reasons why ether and chloroform were to be adopted in its stead as preferred surgical anesthetics.

Not only were ether and chloroform more potent anesthetics than nitrous oxide, but they were also available as liquids. While relatively complex apparatus was essential for administration of a gas such as nitrous oxide, the equipment required to deliver ether or chloroform anesthesia proved remarkably simple. A very common practice was to pour the liquid anesthetic directly from the bottle on to a sponge or folded handkerchief placed over the patient's face where it quickly vaporized. In fact, only two basic requirements were necessary to administer these inhalation anesthetics; i.e., a "rag and a bottle" (Figures 1-1 and 1-2).

Although the patient received an adequate amount of vaporized anesthetic with this simple approach, openness of the technique could not help but dissipate large amounts of waste anesthetic gas into the surrounding atmosphere. The extent of anesthetic pollution must have been readily apparent to all, since little more than a sense of smell was necessary to define its presence. Surprisingly, although high levels

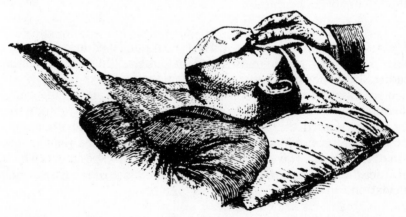

Figure 1-1 Simpson's method for administering chloroform on the corner of a towel. (From K.D. Thomas, *The Development of Anaesthesia Apparatus,* London: Blackwell Scientific Publications, 1975. Reprinted by permission of the author.)

of anesthetic pollution were obviously recognizable, their presence generated little attention, and only modest concerns were raised in terms of the unavoidable rebreathing of these omnipresent anesthetic vapors.

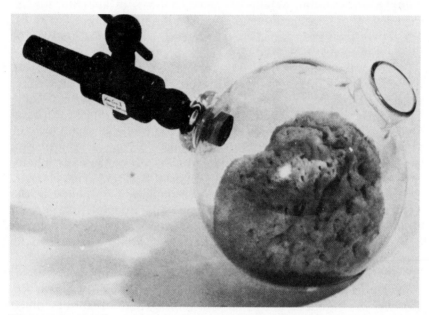

Figure 1-2 Replica of Morton's ether inhaler. (From K.D. Thomas, *The Development of Anaesthesia Apparatus,* London: Blackwell Scientific Publications, 1975. Reprinted by permission of the author.)

There were, however, a few serious problems. A number of exposed individuals (doctors and nurses) were adversely affected by the waste anesthetic gases and developed symptoms of headache, weakness, dizziness and loss of appetite. Kirschner (1925), in a report of operating room hygiene, ascribed weakness and headaches sometimes noted in surgeons to be related to "acute poisoning from long inhalations of air filled with narcotic vapors." Perthes (1925) offered a similar explanation for the occurrence of acute and chronic cardiac conditions.

Julius Hirsch and Adolf Kappurs (1929), working at the Institute for Hygiene in Berlin, subsequently published a damaging report regarding problems of anesthetic air pollution in the operating room and noted that "the inhalations of anesthetic agents present in the air of the operating room have an injurious effect on the health of surgeons and those who assist them. Whereas acute toxicity is unlikely, chronic toxicity cannot be excluded."

Werthmann (1948) first noted the phenomenon of "chronic ether intoxication" describing in detail the symptoms present in three individuals working for long periods in operating rooms where ether anesthesia was in frequent use. These workers evidenced multiple complaints, including weakness, headache, loss of appetite, loss of memory, poor concentrating ability, and inflammation of the gums. Objective findings included lymphocytosis, eosinophilia, and minor changes in the electrocardiogram.

To complicate the situation further, additional concerns were later introduced, including the suggestion of increased risks of sterility, nephritis, and asthma (Davis, 1968). In these cases, the claimants made strong arguments for a causative association of their individual health problems with exposure to waste anesthetic gas. Foregger (1944), in his eulogy of Dr. Gwathmey, wrote; "Gwathmey's disease—asthma—might be considered an effect of the daily inhalation of ether vapors during the many years of his life... [The] effect of ether as a solvent of lipoids may prove similarly detrimental to the tissues of the lungs...producing a drying and hardening process with resultant shrinkage. If ether irritated the lungs of the patient, as it was held to do, why should not prolonged exposure produce damage to the lungs of the anesthetist?"

Another example of the developing awareness and concern was provided in a report which appeared in the first issue of *Current Researches in Anesthesia and Analgesia* (Anonymous, 1922) describing the death of the anesthetist Dr. Edward Costain. In his writings, the biographer portrayed Dr. Costain as "a martyr to his skill who paid with his life for his humane work." On his deathbed, Dr. Costain was said to have expressed the wish that "the public be not informed of his death when it occurred, lest the medical profession suffer a blow, when it became known that the administration of anesthetics had cost the life of a man who had spared the suffering of more than 30,000 people undergoing operation."

Although relatively few individuals were concerned about occupational exposure of anesthetists in such seriously detrimental health terms, definite efforts were made to decrease exposure and improve the potentially unhealthful situation. Over the years, specialized types of anesthetic apparatus were designed to reduce waste anesthetic pollution. One of the first pieces of scientifically designed equipment for the control of operating room anesthetic pollution was developed by Kelling (1918, 1922). In this system, a close-fitting mask, which contained a small inlet tube for administration of the vaporized ether or chloroform, was placed on the patient's face. The outlet tube, with nonrebreathing valve and rubber bag, was in turn exhausted to the ventilating chimney of the operating room (Figure 1-3). A more sophisticated variant of an anesthetic gas scavenging machine was later developed by Perthes (1925). Containing a powerful electric motor, this apparatus removed waste gases from the area of the patient's head by suction and then transferred these gases via a long conduit in the floor to outside the operating room (Figure 1-4).

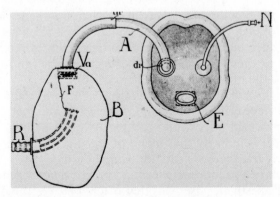

Figure 1-3 Mask for removal of waste anesthetic vapors. **N**—inlet for ether or chloroform vapor; **E**—inlet for room air inhalation; **A**—exhalation tube; **Va**—nonrebreathing valve; **R**—outlet to ventilating chimney. (From G. Kelling, *Zentralbl Chir.*, 45:602–606, 1918. Reprinted by permission of the publisher.)

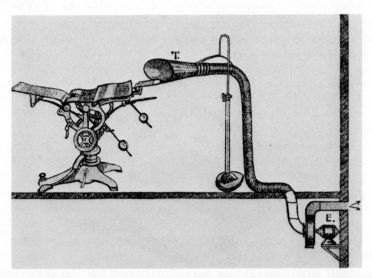

Figure 1-4 Early gas scavenging device. Gas was suctioned away from the head of the patient and transferred outside the operating room. (From G. Perthes, *Zentralbl Chir.*, 52:852–854, 1925. Reprinted by permission of the publisher.)

6

An interesting variant to this scavenging approach was provided by Wieloch (1925), who utilized a pillowlike metal box which had an indentation for the patient's head. The indentation was in turn surrounded by a number of escape holes through which the excess narcotic vapors were vacuumed into a drain tube leading to the exhauster (Figure 1-5).

Yet another method for removal of waste anesthetic gases was suggested by Holscher (1928), who located a carbon-silica gel filter above the applied face mask. These chemical adsorbents served to trap exhaled gases as they left the patient's lungs and before they could be released into the operating room (Figure 1-6).

Although each of these various approaches was claimed by the inventor to achieve efficient removal of the waste anesthetic gases, most were so impractical in cost and complexity as to be unacceptable for clinical use. It is unlikely that many of the described pieces of equipment actually left the inventors' drawing boards.

Undoubtedly, a more efficient and practical approach for removal of the waste anesthetic gases was that offered by Werthmann (1948) in his concept of an "artificial climate" within the operating room. As described by Werthmann, the basic requirements included a vacuuming suction placed at floor level to pull out the heavy anesthetic vapors, and a fresh-air inflow from the ceiling toward the floor. In this way, the gases were thought to be removed without recirculation and without dispersing floor contaminants, such as bacteria and dust. The practicality of Werthmann's approach was established by reported improvement in health and efficiency of operating room personnel following installation of this device.

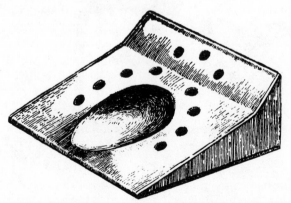

Figure 1-5 Metal pillow box for removal of waste anesthetic vapors. Heavier anesthetic gases passed through collection ports and were directed into a common outflow tube for disposal. (From J. Wieloch, *Zentralbl Gynaekol.,* 49:2768–2771, 1925. Reprinted by permission of the publisher.)

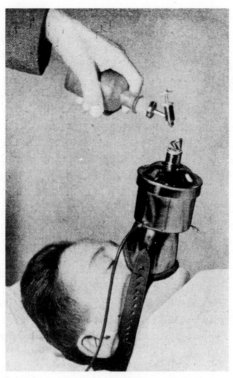

Figure 1-6   Mask filter for removal of waste anesthetic vapors. Exhaled air was adsorbed by a charcoal-silica gel mixture. (From Holscher, *Zentralbl Chir.,* 55:1161–1162, 1928. Reprinted by permission of the publisher.)

Despite the wide variety of mechanical methods developed for its control, and written concerns regarding its presence, anesthetic gas pollution in the operating room succeeded in generating only modest levels of attention. A dramatic awakening, however, finally occurred in the wake of a report published by Vaisman (1967). This study described in considerable detail the adverse working conditions and associated health problems present among Russian anesthetists. Vaisman's report was soon followed by other studies which confirmed the presence of similar health problems in anesthetists elsewhere in the world. These studies rapidly led to a worldwide interest and concern. As evidence, the past decade has seen some 20 epidemiologic surveys in eight countries and in excess of 300 published reports involving problems associated with waste anesthetics. Although there exists no absolute proof for a causal relationship between these waste anesthetics and the health of occupationally exposed personnel, strong evidence supporting this association continues to accumulate.

REFERENCES

Anonymous. Noted anesthetist dies a martyr to his skill. *Anesth Analg. (Cleve)* 1:18, 1922.

Davis, D.A. The operating room: an unhealthy environment? Edited by D.A. Davis. In *Historical Vignettes of Modern Anesthesia.* Philadelphia: F.A. Davis Co., 1968.

Davy, Humphrey. *Researches, Chemical and Philosophical, Chiefly Concerning Nitrous Oxide, or Dephlogisticated Nitrous Air and Its Respiration.* London: J. Johnson, 1800.

Foregger, R. Gwathmey. *Anesthesiology.* 5:296–299, 1944.

Hirsch, J.B., and Kappurs, A.L. Uber die mengen des narkoseathers in der luft von operationsaaslen. *Z Hyg.* 110:391–398, 1929.

Holscher, F. Zur erwarmung der narkosegase. *Zentralbl Chir.* 55:1161–1162, 1928.

Kelling, G. Uber die beseitigung der narkosedampfe aus dem operationsaale. *Zentralbl Chir.* 45:602–606, 1918.

_____. Narkosemaske zur selbsttatigen abfuhrung der chloroform und ather dampfe. *Zentralbl Chir.* 29:1046–1066, 1922.

Kirschner, M. Zur hygiene des operationssaales. *Zentralbl Chir.* 52:2162–2165, 1925.

Perthes, G. Shutz der am operationstisch beschaftigten vor schadigung durch die narkosegase. *Zentralbl Chir.* 52:852–854, 1925.

Vaisman, A.I. Working conditions in surgery and their effect on health of anesthesiologists. *Eksp Khir Anestheziol.* 3:44–49, 1967.

Wells, H. A history of the discovery of the application of nitrous oxide gas, ether, and other vapors, to surgical operations. Hartford, Conn.: J.G. Wells, 1847.

Werthmann, H. Beitrag zur chronischen atherintoxikation der chirurgen. *Beitr Klin Chir.* 178:149–156, 1948.

Wieloch, J. Zur beseitigung der narkosedampfe aus dem operationssaal. *Zentralbl Gynaekol.* 49:2768–2770, 1925.

2 Levels of Exposure to Trace Anesthetic Gases

Charles E. Whitcher

The concentrations of trace anesthetic gases inhaled by personnel who work in anesthetizing and postanesthetic recovery locations are of interest. Assuming a causal relationship between reported occupational disease and the waste anesthetic gases, concentrations of the latter would relate quantitatively to disease incidence. This relationship is supported by data indicating a diminishing disease rate associated with various levels of anesthetic exposure among groups of operating room personnel, i.e., physician anesthetists, nurse anesthetists, operating room nurses, and operating room technicians (Cohen et al., 1974). A crude dose-response relationship constructed with these data could prove useful in predicting specific exposure levels required to achieve acceptable reductions in disease incidence. Measured gas concentrations would thus indicate the position of a particular exposed population on the dose-response curve and also document effectiveness of the control effort.

Recently, many of the factors which affect inhaled waste gas concentrations and their measurement have been recognized. Unfortunately, much of the earlier reported data were acquired under inadequately defined conditions and must be interpreted with caution.

FACTORS THAT AFFECT WASTE GAS CONCENTRATIONS

Factors that affect waste anesthetic gas concentrations can be separated into several categories, including the air conditioning system, anesthetic gas flow rates, anesthetizing techniques, anesthetic equipment leakage, and sampling methods.

Air Conditioning System

The important role of the air conditioning system in the distribution and elimination of waste gases will be discussed in detail in a later chapter (Chapter 6) and is mentioned here for cohesiveness. The air conditioning system provides an inflow of air usually sufficient to cause thorough mixing of all anesthetic gases released into the room. Mixtures of gases released into the room remain mixed, and the heavier gases do not settle (Whitcher, Cohen, and Trudell 1971). Mixing, however, is often imperfect, and localized areas of anesthetic concentration above and below the average for the room ("hot spots" and "cold spots") are apt to occur. It is apparent that gas samples obtained in close proximity to personnel are those most apt to represent the anesthetic gas concentrations inhaled.

Figure 2-1 suggests the stirring effect produced by the air conditioning system. Marked variations in concentration can be introduced by the location of furniture, drapes, and personnel. Table 2-1 indicates distribution patterns for nitrous oxide (N_2O) and halothane measured in two operating rooms. Note that anesthetic concentrations are similar whether measured or calculated.

Anesthetic Gas Flowrate

In the absence of scavenging, flowrates of fresh anesthetic gases in the anesthesia machine have significant impact on the concentrations present in room air. The higher the flowrates, the greater the levels of room concentration. With efficient gas scavenging, flowrates have only a minor influence on anesthetic gas concentrations.

Anesthetizing Techniques

The pediatric anesthetist who induces anesthesia with the gravitation technique receives, and provides to others, a heavy anesthetic exposure. The same is true of the anesthetist who begins flow of the anesthetic gases prior to application of the face mask. Thoughtful attention to technical details listed in Chapter 6 may help significantly in reducing anesthetic concentrations inhaled by personnel.

Anesthetic Equipment Leakage

Leaky equipment inevitably increases occupational exposure. For example, a leak in the high-pressure nitrous oxide line leading to the gas machine may be sufficient to obscure any reduction in exposure achieved by scavenging. During the early development of control measures, automatic patient ventilators with scavenging facilities were not available. Scavenging devices themselves, whether purchased or fabricated locally, are not necessarily gas-tight. Multiple and diverse sources of gas leakage are possible, as suggested in Figure 2-2. Extraneous leak sources thus can heavily pollute a room that does not even contain a gas machine.

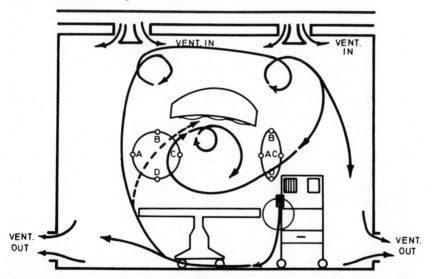

Figure 2-1 Smoke distribution patterns in an air conditioned operating room. High concentration (hot spot) occurred beneath light. A,B, etc. indicate gas measurement (From O. Berner. *Acta Anaesthesiol Scand.*, 22:44–54, 1978) Reprinted by permission of Munksgaard International Publishers.

Table 2-1
Observed Average Concentrations of Anesthetic Gases in Operating and Delivery Rooms

Test	Height 220 cm			Height 140 cm			Height 2 cm		
	N_2O (ppm)	Halothane (ppm)	$N_2O/$ Halothane	N_2O (ppm)	Halothane (ppm)	$N_2O/$ Halothane	N_2O (ppm)	Halothane (ppm)	$N_2O/$ Halothane
1 (Delivery room)	113 ± 49	1.80 ± 0.72	63 ± 3	119 ± 22	1.88 ± 0.41	64 ± 2	116 ± 25	1.76 ± 0.35	66 ± 2
2 (Delivery room)	100 ± 13	1.76 ± 0.27	57 ± 4	106 ± 18	1.94 ± 0.35	58 ± 2	110 ± 14	2.00 ± 0.25	55 ± 1
3 (Delivery room)	104 ± 46	1.54 ± 0.40	62 ± 4	114 ± 66	2.11 ± 0.99	53 ± 4	130 ± 24	2.06 ± 0.41	64 ± 4
4 (Operating room)	71 ± 11	1.08 ± 0.14	65 ± 4	143 ± 107	2.53 ± 1.81	56 ± 3	97 ± 20	1.66 ± 0.34	59 ± 3

Test Conditions and Calculated Concentrations

Test	Air Conditioning Flow (ft^3/min)	Room Changes/hr	Height of Anesthetic Gas Source (cm)	Anesthetic Gas Flow (L/min)		Ratio of Flowrates $N_2O/$ Halothane	Expected Average Concentrations (ppm)	
				N_2O	Halothane		N_2O	Halothane
1	1000	21.3	92	3.0	0.050	60	106	1.77
2	1000	21.3	2	3.0	0.050	60	106	1.77
3	450	10.1	92	3.0	0.050	60	238	3.93
4	1200	19.5	92	3.0	0.050	60	88	1.47

Source: Piziali et al., *Anesthesiology* 45:487–494, 1976. Reprinted by permission of the publisher.

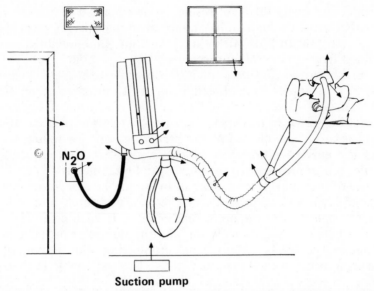

Figure 2-2 Sources of N₂O in occupational exposure. Arrows indicate leakages frequently found. Pollution may occur independent of room activities. (From Whitcher et al., *J Am Dent Assoc.* 95:763–776, 1977.)

Sampling Methods

Sampling methods have a marked influence on reported gas concentrations. A significant problem in gas sampling is that concentrations of anesthetic gases in the room air frequently are not static but are subject to localized areas of marked and rapid variation (Figure 2-3). (A dramatic example of a serious sampling problem which demonstrates the influence of anesthetic equipment and technique is seen in the gas leakage pattern displayed in the frontispiece.)

It is notable that a small nitrous oxide leak in the high-pressure system, insufficient to cause a perceptible increase in the average concentration in room air, may measure 1 million ppm at its source. Unfortunately, the anesthetist immediately downwind of such a leak might inhale high concentrations far beyond expectations based on the average measured room concentration. These considerations underscore the desirability of sampling as close as possible to the breathing zone.

Wide variations in individual measurements of gas concentrations lead to the common practice of averaging, or time-weighting. The extent of averaging may be critical in that too much or too little averaging may yield misleading results and mask the relevant data.

14

Consider the vastly different results to be obtained in grab samples secured at either the high- or low-concentration peaks shown in Figure 2-3 compared with those from an eight-hour, time-weighted sample obtained from an operating room used only one hour.

An important consideration is the objective to be met in measurement of air samples. One objective may be to measure occupational exposure, and a second objective may be to measure efficiency of control measures. In the first case, samples relevant to occupational exposure are best collected at the breathing zone. Sampling should cover the entire workday, or at least a significantly representative sample. It is appropriate to continue sampling even during periods of absence of personnel from the room. In the second case, measurement of the efficiency of control measures can be accurately assessed only when the anesthetic gases are actually in use. In such measurements, the time between cases is irrelevant and should not be included in the sampling process. For routine air monitoring, the desirability of measuring occupational exposure per se is questionable in that safe

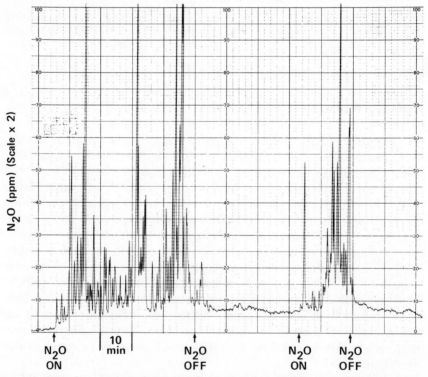

Figure 2-3 Variations in N_2O concentrations measured in the breathing zone of the dentist over a 120-minute sampling period. (From Whitcher et al. *J Am Dent Assoc.* 95:763–776, 1977)

levels of anesthetic exposure have not been identified. We are advised to maintain the lowest reasonably achievable concentrations.

End-tidal, rebreathing, and blood samples obtained under carefully controlled circumstances can accurately reflect occupational exposure, but the inconveniences of these methods have led to the more widespread use of breathing zone, work zone, and general area sampling.

ANESTHETIC GAS CONCENTRATIONS
IN THE OPERATING ROOM

The published literature on anesthetic gas concentrations in room air of the anesthetizing and recovery areas will be reviewed with the intent of offering a representative sample of available work. One of the earliest studies of occupational exposure in the operating room was published by Linde and Bruce (1969). This work was conducted in two hospitals with a total of 21 individual operating rooms in which the air conditioning systems provided 12 nonrecirculating air exchanges per hour. High-flow anesthetic techniques were used. The overall average anesthetic concentrations were nitrous oxide 130 ppm and halothane 10 ppm. In this study, end-tidal and room concentrations of halothane did not correlate consistently. The higher end-tidal samples reflect recent higher exposure typical of breathing zone samples.

Hallén, Ehrner-Samuel, and Thomason (1970) reported halothane concentrations employing nonrebreathing techniques in an air conditioned operating room. Air samples were obtained in the breathing zone of the anesthetist. Total gas flow was 5 to 6 L/min. Mean halothane concentration measured at a sampling site farther than 25 cm from the anesthetist's head was 8 ppm. Much higher concentrations were found at sampling sites less than 25 cm from the anesthetist. Expired air of the anesthetist examined by a rebreathing technique contained a mean concentration of halothane of 5.2 ppm.

Distribution of halothane in the operating room air was investigated by Whitcher et al. (1971). A total of 329 samples were obtained in 13 test locations, 9 of which were close to or within the anesthetist's breathing zone. The air conditioning system was nonrecirculating with an air exchange rate approximating 10 per hour. With a nonrebreathing system, employed at a flowrate of 10 L/min, the highest mean halothane concentration (12.88 ppm) was found in the absence of scavenging at a site close to the exhaust of the nonrebreathing valve. Away from this leak source, mean halothane concentrations were lower (approximately 2 ppm) and more evenly distributed. A circle carbon dioxide absorption system employed at flowrates of 4 to 5 L/min in the absence of scavenging yielded a maximum mean halothane concentration of 9 ppm at a site close to the adjustable relief valve, and 0.6 to 1.6 ppm in more remote locations. Results following scavenging are summarized in Table 2-2. Except for sampling sites close to the carbon dioxide absorber, concentrations were similar throughout the room regardless of sampling site. Scavenging achieved approximately a 90% reduction in concentration.

Further studies collected end-tidal gas samples in a group of operating nurses and anesthetists. At the end of the workday, samples from the nurses and anesthetists contained mean halothane concentrations of 0.21 ± 0.04 ppm and 0.46 ± 0.07 ppm, respectively. These data confirm the suspected lower exposure of the operating room nurse compared to the anesthetist.

Whitcher et al. (1975) reported results of 202 grab samples of nitrous oxide in room air at various sites in 14 operating rooms. Samples were obtained regardless of room activities. The air conditioning systems exchanged fresh air 12 to 18 times per hour. Results were similar in all sites sampled, with concentrations measuring 13 to 18 ppm (Table 2-3).

A sampling technique described by Davenport et al. (1976) consists of collection of nitrous oxide and halothane in evacuated glass bottles carried by personnel. A negative pressure was maintained in the bottles, and samples continuously aspirated by a catheter terminating near the anesthetist's nose. During a three-hour sampling period, without control measures, mean and range values for nitrous oxide were 269 ppm (range 108 to 430 ppm), and for halothane 3.6

Table 2-2
Halothane (ppm) at Selected Sampling Sites
Conditions include scavenging and nonrecirculating air conditioning. (Halothane 1%, in 4 to 5 L/min of diluent gases.)

	Sampling Site		Horizontal Distance from Relief Valve*	
Floor	*Ceiling*	*Grille*	*3 ft*	*1 ft*
0.47 ± 0.09	0.40 ± 0.09	0.44 ± 0.11	0.62 ± 0.13	2.22 ± 0.37

Source: Whitcher et al., *Anesthesiology* 35:348–353, 1971.
*All samples measured 3 ft above floor ($n = 11$ for each site.)

ppm (range 1.0 to 8.0 ppm) (Table 2-4). Control measures were subsequently introduced in two stages. The first stage consisted of the addition of a "banjo" fitting which served to direct waste gas flow away from the anesthetist. The second stage consisted of the attachment of this same fitting to suction. With the "banjo" fitting alone, breathing zone concentrations were only slightly reduced, to 243 (range 73 to 400) ppm nitrous oxide and 1.1 (range 0 to 3.4) ppm halothane. With the "banjo" fitting attached to suction, nitrous oxide was reduced to 127 (range 67.5 to 225) ppm and halothane to 0.57 (range 0 to 1.6) ppm.

Further studies were conducted in which results of 10-minute sampling periods were compared in both induction and operating rooms. The short sampling period insured the anesthetist's presence

Table 2-3
Concentrations of N_2O (ppm) at Various Sites
in 14 Air Conditioned Operating Rooms

Sampling Site					
Grille	Anesthetist	Surgeon	Scrub Nurse	Circulating Nurse	Door
15 ± 2.7	18 ± 2.9	17 ± 5.0	13 ± 3.2	14 ± 2.8	14 ± 2.8

Source: Whitcher et al. U.S. Government Printing Office, 1975.

Table 2-4
Results of Integrated Personal Sampling,
Showing Means and Ranges
Exposure to anesthetists was over a three-hour operating session.

	N_2O (ppm)	Halothane (ppm)
No precautions ($n = 8$)	269 (108–430)	3.6 (1.0–8.0)
"Banjo" fitting ($n = 11$)	243 (73–400)	1.1 (0–3.4)
Scavenging ($n = 13$)	127 (67.5–225)	0.57 (0–1.6)

Source: Davenport et al., *Br Med J.* 2:1219–1220, 1976. Reprinted by permission of the publisher.

throughout sampling; as a result, concentrations were higher than in the three-hour collected samples (Table 2-5). The average exposure of the anesthetist was more than twice that expected from indicated gas volumes released from the anesthesia machine and cleared by the air conditioning system. This result could be explained by extraneous leak sources.

Göthe, Ovrum, and Hallén (1976) reported halothane and ethanol concentrations in nine suites in six different hospitals. A total of 310 time-weighted samples were obtained in the breathing zone and general work zone. Results further confirmed the higher exposure of anesthetic nurses compared to surgical nurses, and indicated higher concentrations during anesthesia by face mask compared to endotracheal techniques. Halothane concentrations in all categories ranged from mean values of 2.2 to 10.4 ppm. A reduction of halothane concentration followed increased room ventilation.

Berner (1978) reported nitrous oxide and halothane concentrations measured in the breathing zones of anesthetists and operating room nurses. The air conditioning system provided 20 fresh air exchanges per hour. Distribution of anesthetic gases was studied by releasing smoke into the room. Using leak-proof anesthetic systems with scavenging, the average concentration of halothane in the anesthetist's breathing zone was 0.02 ppm, and the average concentration inhaled by the nurse was 0.01 ppm. Comparable studies in which nitrous oxide concentrations were measured yielded mean concentrations below 2 to 3 ppm for both the anesthetist and the nurse. These results are among the lowest concentrations reported in the literature. Our own work confirms the possibility of maintaining such concentrations under rigidly controlled conditions (Whitcher et al., 1975).

Beynen, Knapp, and Rehder (1978) reported a series of end-tidal samples and grab samples obtained from a sampling site behind the anesthetist's head. Nitrous oxide flowrates were 0.7 to 7.0 L/min. In an operating room under experimental conditions with no surgery in progress and with scavenging, nitrous oxide concentrations measured in end-tidal and grab samples were highly correlated. Similar comparisons during surgery yielded inconsistent correlation. It might be expected that single grab samples, which are not time-weighted, would under certain circumstances correlate poorly with end-tidal samples, which are inherently time-weighted. It would also be expected that the increasing average concentration of nitrous oxide (22, 63, and 144 ppm) noted in the three rooms tested in the "scavenger functioning" group would associate inversely with the decreasing fresh-air flow from the air conditioning system.

Korttila, Pfäffli, and Ertama (1978) studied concentrations of nitrous oxide in the room air, blood, and end-tidal air of 10 operating room nurses. The operating rooms were air conditioned at a fresh-air

Table 2-5
Exposure Levels of One Anesthetist Repeated over 10-Minute Sampling Periods
Magill circuit, spontaneous respiration with N_2O: O_2 at 6:3 L/min, halothane at 2%.

	Anesthesia Induction Room		Operating Room	
	N_2O (ppm)	Halothane (ppm)	N_2O (ppm)	Halothane (ppm)
No precautions taken				
No. samples	8	8	5	4
Mean	3038	52.1	453	5.3
(Range)	(600–5380)	(12.5–115.0)	(301–630)	(4.0–6.3)
"Banjo" fitting				
No. samples	8	8	10	10
Mean	887	12.7	250	2.45
(Range)	(450–1323)	(8.1–17.1)	(25–464)	(0–4.3)
Scavenging				
No. samples	6	6	12	12
Mean	152	3.1	62.0	0.46
(Range)	(67.5–235)	(0.75–8.5)	(0–147)	(0–1.25)

Source: Davenport et al., *Br Med J.* 2:1219–1220, 1976. Reprinted by permission of the publisher.

exchange rate of approximately 10 per hour. The nurses worked approximately three hours in one of three operating rooms. The breathing system was semiopen, and scavenging was not practiced. Bag samples of room air were collected during consecutive periods of one-half to one hour using a battery-powered sampling pump in a fixed sampling site located between the anesthetist and the instrument nurse. Air sampling began with induction of anesthesia and ended 15 minutes after the end of the last anesthetic. End-tidal samples were obtained 15 to 60 minutes after leaving the operating room. During anesthetic administration, nitrous oxide concentrations in room air were 380 ± 57 ppm, and end-tidal samples measured 153 ± 111 ppm. Correlation of these values is poor, and may be explained by the delay in obtaining end-tidal samples.

Results from a commercial testing laboratory,[1] in which subscribers reported that scavenging was practiced and sample collection protocol followed, indicate that in 124 samples of nitrous oxide the mean concentration was 56 ppm. Sixty-nine of the samples contained less than 25 ppm nitrous oxide. Halothane concentrations reported in 28 samples averaged 0.64 ppm, with 14 samples measuring less than 0.5 ppm. Enflurane measured in 33 cases was reported as 1.32 ppm, with 32 samples showing less than 1 ppm. A second laboratory[2] reported that in 130 samples with control measures unspecified, a mean concentration of nitrous oxide was 194 ppm, with 59 samples measuring less than 25 ppm. Halothane concentrations in 48 measurements yielded a mean value of 13 ppm, with 24 samples measuring less than 0.5 ppm. Enflurane in 32 samples was reported at a mean concentration of 4.9 ppm, and only 3 samples were reported at less than 1 ppm. Interpretation of these results must be guarded because many circumstances of sampling were beyond control of the testing laboratory. Nevertheless, it is apparent that concentrations of many of the samples reported were considerably above suggested NIOSH standards.

A study of gas concentrations measured during surgery in the operating suite of a large general teaching hospital has recently been completed (Whitcher et al., unpublished data). The air conditioning system was nonrecirculating with an exchange rate averaging 15 fresh-air changes per hour. Anesthetic equipment received quarterly preventive maintenance performed by the manufacturer's representative or equivalent. Anesthetists included private practitioners, full-time faculty, and residents. The infrared analyzer[3] designed for simul-

---

[1]Boehringer Laboratories, Inc., Wynnewood, Pennsylvania.
[2]Air Test Labs, Inc., Rochester, New York
[3]Wilks Model 80, Foxboro-Wilks, East Norwalk, Connecticut.

taneous measurement of several gases was zeroed with air in an area known to be free of anesthetic agents. Span calibration was verified by use of custom-mixed standard gases. The analyzer, operating on battery power, was moved into each of the 11 rooms under test in random sequence, with sampling rounds conducted each working hour of the day shift. To date approximately 190 individual samples have been collected within the breathing zones of the anesthetists, circulating nurses, and scrub nurses. Samples were collected over a 30-second period. The sampling site was as close as practical to the breathing zones of the anesthetist, scrub nurse, and circulating nurse. Where the circulating nurse was inaccessible, the surgeon was substituted. Whenever possible, the breathing zone utilized was the midpoint of the clavicle; otherwise, the lateral aspect of the neck was used (Table 2-6).

Table 2-6
Concentrations (ppm) of N_2O in Breathing Zone
Studies conducted in 11 air conditioned operating rooms with anesthesia in progress.

		Anesthetist	Circulating Nurse	Scrub Nurse
A.	Mask + Endotracheal Technique:			
	Mean ± SE	50 ± 6.5	29 ± 3.6	30 ± 3.8
	Range	1 – 400	1 – 230	1 –310
	n	190	190	190
	%ppm<25; (>100)	69(26)	74(19)	73(9)
B.	Mask Technique:			
	Mean ± SE	180 ± 25	100 ± 14	100 ± 14
	Range	23 – 430	9 – 230	9 – 250
	n	26	25	26
	%ppm<25; (>100)	4(62)	8(44)	8(42)
C.	Endotracheal Technique:			
	Mean ± SE	16 ± 5	9 ± 2	8 ± 1
	Range	12 – 370	0.5 – 80	0.5 – 69
	n	72	71	70
	%ppm<25; (>100)	93(1)	95(0)	97(0)

Source: C.E. Whitcher and L.V.M. Siukola, (*Anesthesiology,* in press).

Mean nitrous oxide concentrations shown in Table 2-6 were obtained during anesthetic administration, irrespective of the anesthetic technique used. Values averaged 50 ± 7, 29 ± 4, and 30 ± 4 ppm N_2O for the anesthestist, circulating nurse and scrub nurse, respectively. Data obtained during exclusive use of a face mask indicated N_2O concentrations (ppm) of 181 ± 25, 105 ± 14, and 102 ± 14, respectively. When supplemented by an endotracheal technique, the respective concentrations were 16 ± 5, 9 ± 2, and 8 ± 1 ppm. Still lower concentrations would be expected by exclusion of cases induced with inhalation agents via a face mask and subsequently intubated.

Higher concentrations of N_2O found in the present study compared to a previous report by the same authors (Whitcher et al., 1975) are likely accounted for by the fact that earlier study samples were obtained regardless of operating room activities and included rooms using local anesthetics or temporarily empty.

We conclude that substantial risks of anesthetic exposure, and high levels frequently prevailing during the use of the face mask, increase the indications for anesthetic administration by endotracheal tube.

ANESTHETIC GAS CONCENTRATIONS IN THE RECOVERY ROOM

Bruce and Linde (1972) reported personnel samples obtained from recovery room nurses in two different hospitals. Mean concentrations of halothane were 0.36 ppm and 0.61 ppm, respectively.

Pfäffli, Nikki, and Ahlman (1972) reported concentrations of nitrous oxide and halothane in three recovery rooms. Conditions were not completely described, but concentrations were surprisingly high, with mean nitrous oxide measurements of 305 ppm (range 20 to 1660 ppm) and halothane 3.0 ppm (range 0.9 to 8.2 ppm).

Davenport et al. (1976) briefly mention studies of recovery room nurses using time-weighted sampling equipment (vacuum bottles), all samples obtained in the breathing zone. Concentrations of nitrous oxide were 18 ppm (range 15 to 25 ppm) and halothane 0.1 ppm (range 0 to 0.5 ppm).

Berner (1978b) reported results obtained in three recovery rooms based on grab sampling methods with 108 analyses. Nitrous oxide concentrations were measured in locations usually frequented by the nurse. "Actual exposure" was 10, 32, and 34 ppm, calculated on the basis of measured concentrations, estimated time spent in each location, and the fresh-air exchange rate of the air conditioning system expressed in terms of cubic meters of fresh air per patient per hour (Table 2-7).

Table 2-7
Average and Range of N$_2$O Concentrations in Three Differently Ventilated Recovery Rooms
Ventilation was nonrecirculating. Average N$_2$O concentration is calculated on the basis of time spent by the personnel in measuring areas.

Room Ventilation (m³/patient/h)	Average N$_2$O Concentration (ppm)				No. Samples
	50 cm above Thorax	Foot End of Bed 120 cm above Floor	2 m. from Bed, 180 cm above Floor	Calculated N$_2$O Mean Concentration	
500	29 (0–100)	3 (0–12)	1.5 (0–12)	10	33
200	78 (10–270)	14 (0–50)	13 (0–50)	32	39
150	68 (5–280)	18 (0–50)	18 (0–50)	34	36

Source: Berner, *Acta Anaesth Scand.* 22:55–57, 1978b. Reprinted by permission of Munksgaard International Publishers.

Korttila et al. (1978) compared nitrous oxide concentrations in room air with end-tidal air of recovery room nurses. Sampling techniques consisted of three consecutive one-hour periods of sampling using a battery-powered pump with storage of samples in gas-tight bags. The precise sampling site is not mentioned, but it may be presumed that samples were obtained within or close to the breathing zones of personnel. Room air inhaled by the nurses contained a surprisingly high concentration of nitrous oxide, 100 ± 21 ppm (range 79 to 125 ppm). Low air conditioning flowrates for the recovery room, not specifically mentioned, could explain the high values reported.

Comprehensive studies of anesthetic concentrations in the recovery room remain to be done. However, published information, considered with our own unpublished results, confirm that in recovery areas with adequate air conditioning, personnel are probably exposed to concentrations lower than those in clean operating rooms.

ANESTHETIC GAS EXPOSURE IN THE DENTAL OPERATORY

It might be expected that the dentist who employs anesthetic/ analgesic gases such as nitrous oxide would be subject to high exposure levels and that comparable exposures would be shared by his assistants. The nasal mask employed in gas administration is often loosely applied and favors leakage. Furthermore, anesthetic equipment is frequently less well maintained in the dental operatory than in the hospital, and the air conditioning system, when present, is often a recirculating unit.

Millard and Corbett (1974) reported nitrous oxide concentrations measured during operative dental procedures. The N_2O flowrate was 4 L/min into the nasal mask. Samples were obtained at 15-minute intervals in gas-tight syringes at a site two inches in front of the nose of the dentist and his assistant. Concentrations indicate a range of 3800 to 6800 ppm nitrous oxide in the area of the dentist. For the assistant, mean values were 1900 to 5900 ppm nitrous oxide.

Scheidt, Stanford, and Ayer (1977), working in a single dental operatory, measured nitrous oxide concentrations during simulated dentistry in four subjects under nitrous oxide analgesia. Conditions included an absence of ventilation and a nitrous oxide flowrate of 1800 ml/min. A tightly fitted nasal mask with a one-way valve excluded room air on inhalation and permitted exhalation into the room. Operatory air samples were obtained over a period of 30 seconds at intervals of 5, 15, 30, and 45 minutes at various distances from the relief valve of the nosepiece and at various angles from the main pathway of the exhaust gases. Samples obtained at angles of 90° and 180° and from distances of 1 to 2 feet would approximate the breathing zones of the dentist and his assistant. Sixteen data points which met these criteria yielded a mean nitrous oxide concentration of 920 ppm (range 220 to 1600 ppm). This publication elucidates several important factors which affect occupational anesthetic exposure in the dental operatory, especially distance and angle of the personnel with respect to the pathway of gases exhaled by the patient and the buildup of concentrations which occurs in the absence of air conditioning.

Swenson (1976) measured halothane and nitrous oxide concentrations during oral surgery in a single operatory. Air samples were obtained during the last general anesthetic of the morning. The nitrous oxide flowrate was 7 L/min. Samples were obtained 15 minutes after the beginning of anesthesia at a point 15 cm horizontal to the patient's nose. Other conditions included use of two different breathing systems and a recirculating air conditioning system. In the absence of control measures, nitrous oxide concentrations averaged 1955 ppm and halothane 33.5 ppm. Scavenging reduced these concentrations to 640 and 6.45 ppm, respectively. Modification of the air conditioning system and outside venting of the effluent from the breathing systems achieved a further reduction of nitrous oxide to 172 ± 77.9 ppm and halothane to 2.25 ± 0.31 ppm. A fitted oropharyngeal pack made of plastic foam was thought to reduce gas leakage from the patient's mouth.

Campbell et al. (1977) measured nitrous oxide and halothane concentrations during oral surgery in three different operatories. Air conditioning is not mentioned, nor are the number of samples and duration of sampling. The breathing system consisted of a nasal inhaler with a mounted exhalation valve utilizing a modified semiopen (Magill) circuit. Samples were obtained at the dentist's headlight and from equivalent locations for the assistants. In a series of 10 patients receiving general anesthesia using 7 L/min of nitrous oxide, the mean concentration of nitrous oxide in the dentist's breathing zone was 2650 ± 70 ppm; the anesthetist's samples contained a mean concentration of 1860 ± 100 ppm; and the assistant's samples contained 2480 ± 11.5 ppm. A second series of patients received nitrous oxide analgesia at a flowrate of 2 L/min. In these four cases, the mean concentration of nitrous oxide inhaled by the dentists was 1000 ppm. The authors noted that the exhaust from the air drill significantly reduced the concentrations of the gas inhaled.

A comprehensive study of nitrous oxide concentration during routine dentistry was reported by Whitcher et al. (1977). A total of 157 time-weighted samples were obtained from three groups of dentists—oral surgeons, pedodontists, and general dentists. Samples were continuously aspirated during nitrous oxide administration from the breathing zones of the dentist and his or her assistant. Results indicate that without control measures (conventional mask), nitrous oxide concentrations measured 900 ± 55 ppm for the dentists and 560 ± 97 ppm for the assistants (Table 2-8). With control measures, which minimized all sources of leakage and further made use of a double-walled nasal scavenging mask, concentrations were reduced by 97%, to 31 ± 2.5 ppm for the dentists and 17 ± 1.7 ppm for the assistants. Use of a concentration-equalizing fan brought the dentists' inhaled concentration to 14 ± 1.5 ppm nitrous oxide. These concentrations in the dental operatory achieved by use of a comprehensive control program (Chapter 6) appear to be the lowest reported.

Allen et al. (1978) reported results obtained with apparatus designed to reduce nitrous oxide exposure in the dental operatory. Air conditioning was not mentioned, but on the basis of previous reports by the same authors, efficient air conditioning probably was present. The use of a modified Mapleson D (Bain) breathing system, with scavenging, achieved mean breathing-zone nitrous oxide concentrations in three dentists of 116 ppm (range 3 to 281 ppm), 32 ppm (range 0 to 192 ppm), and 45 ppm (range 1 to 123 ppm). A tightly fitted nasal mask was used. The methods were evaluated in terms of pressure changes and nitrogen dilution of the anesthetic mixture[5] which might affect patient safety and predictability of analgesia.

Cleaton-Jones et al. (1978) reported studies of nitrous oxide sedation without scavenging in four dental surgeries. Gas samples were obtained at the beginning of the workday and at 30-minute intervals for six hours. Air conditioning was recirculating. The nasal mask was loosely fitted and equipped with an exhaust valve. Nitrous oxide flowrate was 2 to 5 L/min. Not all patients received nitrous oxide, but air samples were obtained regardless. The highest mean breathing zone concentration of nitrous oxide reported (446 ± 702 ppm) occurred in a single room with a dentist using this anesthetic in 23 consecutive patients. The lowest breathing zone concentrations reported were 86 ± 81 ppm, occurring in an operatory in which several dentists worked, but in which the frequency of nitrous oxide use was only 7 patients for the entire workday. These studies reflect occupational exposure to nitrous oxide rather than efficiency of scavenging.

Hannifan, Reist, and Campbell (1978) reported nitrous oxide concentrations without scavenging during oral surgery conducted under general anesthesia and inhalation analgesia. Air conditioning data were not given. Samples were obtained at the dentist's headlight, or at its equivalent for other personnel. In the anesthesia group,

---

[5]Using the currently available double mask introduced in 1977, studies in our laboratories indicate that nitrogen dilution of the anesthetic mixture occurs only as deliberately induced by loosely fitting the mask.

Table 2-8
Studies of Occupational Exposure to N₂O in Dental Operatories of Three Specialities

Categories	No. Dentists	No. Cases	Age (yrs)	Time N₂O on (min)	Mean Flowrates (L/min)		N₂O in Breathing Zone (ppm)	
					N_2O	O_2	Dentist	Assistant
Conventional mask								
General dentists	4	20	30 ± 3.6	31 ± 3.0	2.3 ± 0.13	3.4 ± 0.14	775 ± 63	440 ± 52
Pedodontists	2	17	10 ± 1.1	27 ± 2.9	2.4 ± 0.10	2.9 ± 0.06	940 ± 92	112 ± 23
Oral surgeons	2	15	25 ± 2.4	24 ± 3.1	4.0 ± 0.0	4.0 ± 0.0	1000 ± 130	1600 ± 250
Scavenging mask								
General dentists	4	40	31 ± 1.7	32 ± 2.2	2.6 ± 0.15	2.8 ± 0.09	21 ± 1.9	13 ± 1.3
Pedodontists	2	17	10 ± 0.91	19 ± 1.9	2.4 ± 0.08	2.8 ± 0.06	33 ± 4.0	8.7 ± 3.3
Oral surgeons	2	22	25 ± 2.8	24 ± 2.6	3.6 ± 0.16	3.9 ± 0.17	36 ± 4.1	36 ± 4.4
Scavenging mask and air sweep fan								
General dentist	1	9	11.9 ± 2.7	30 ± 3.8	2.4 ± 0.14	2.7 ± 0.08	15 ± 7.0	11 ± 2.6
Pedodontist	1	9	7.4 ± 1.2	28 ± 4.4	2.3 ± 0.24	3.0 ± 0.0	9.4 ± 0.87	7.5 ± 0.43
Oral surgeon	1	8	24 ± 4.7	37 ± 7.0	4.0 ± 0.0	4.0 ± 0.0	18 ± 3.6	14 ± 2.0
Totals								
Conventional mask	8	52					900 ± 55	560 ± 97
Scavenging mask	8	79					31 ± 2.5	17 ± 1.7
Scavenging mask and fan	3	26					14 ± 1.5	—

Source: Whitcher et al., *J Am Dent Assoc.* 95:763–776, 1977.

nitrous oxide flowrate was 7 L/min. Average inhaled concentrations measured in the breathing zones of the dentist and assistant were 2650 (range 500 to 6000) ppm and 2480 (range 1440 to 5000) ppm, respectively. The analgesia group was managed with nasal masks equipped with a two-way valve intended to allow room-air dilution of the inhaled analgesic gas mixture and to provide an exit route for the exhaled gas mixture. In this group, at a nitrous oxide flowrate of 2 L/min, the mean concentration inhaled by two dentists was 1000 (range 400 to 1540) ppm (Table 2-9). Concentrations of nitrous oxide increased throughout the day, reflecting buildup in the recirculating air conditioning system. In the analgesia group, a considerable difference in average exposure was noted between the anesthetists and assistants. Lowest nitrous oxide concentrations were measured a short distance away from the patient, at the assistant's nose. Concentrations were highest 4 inches from the relief valve. These results again confirm the critical importance of sampling site.

Scaramella et al. (1978) reported studies conducted in a series of 10 air conditioned oral surgical offices. Time-weighted samples were collected in the absence of control measures in gas-tight bags during nitrous oxide administration. The time-weighted samples averaged 158 ± 129 ppm. Additional samples were obtained from the dentist and his two assistants at the end of the surgery by a rebreathing method. The values approximated 210 ± 225 ppm, and within 30 minutes dropped to 22 ppm. These data indicate nitrous oxide concentrations lower than expected. A comparison of the time-weighted breathing zone samples obtained during oral surgery with the rebreathing samples at the end of surgery would be expected to reveal higher concentrations in the perioperative samples. The reverse was reported. Reasons for this discrepancy are not obvious.

As in the operating and recovery rooms, sampling methods used in the dental operatory affect the measured gas concentrations inhaled by personnel. Considering the close proximity of the dental team to significant gas leakage at the patient's head and the high probability of other sources of leakage, a marked variation in reported data is to be expected. It seems reasonable to conclude that during nitrous oxide administration, the dentist frequently breathes as much as 1000 ppm of nitrous oxide, and the assistants as much as 500 ppm. In the dental operatory, where nitrous oxide usage is intermittent or brief, the importance of time-weighted samples must be kept in mind. If the intent is to measure occupational exposure (*not* recommended), the sampling period could cover an entire workday. Such sampling measures applied to a dentist giving few anesthetics, and using *no* control measures, might still meet proposed NIOSH standards. In contrast, measurements obtained during nitrous oxide administration reflect

Table 2-9
Concentrations of N_2O in Dental Operatories

Gas Mixture	Location	Duration (min)	Average Exposure (ppm)	Range of Exposure (ppm)
O_2 (4 L/min); N_2O (2 L/min)	Surgeon	45	400 ± 70	120- 2,660
		75	620 ± 160	80-22,000
		40	1,450 ± 70	280- 4,800
		44	1,540 ± 40	520- 4,800
	Assistant	46	70 ± 16	14- 180
		40	160 ± 11	9- 250
	4 in. from relief valve	—	49,000 ± 1600	13,000-90,000
	Surgeon	22	710 ± 50	350- 5,000
		19	3,000 ± 120	710- 8,500
		36	4,600 ± 90	880-24,000
	Assistant	22	290 ± 27.5	160- 530
		27	380 ± 18	220- 580

Source: Hannifan, Reist, and Campbell, *Am Ind Hyg Assoc J.* 39:69-73, 1978.

the immediate efficiency of the control measures employed. The latter procedure offers maximum protection to personnel.

CONCLUSIONS

An estimate of lowest readily achievable levels suggests nitrous oxide concentration in the operating room of less than 25 ppm and in the dental operatory of less than 50 ppm. These concentrations represent time-weighted samples obtained from the anesthetist's or dentist's breathing zone at a time when anesthetic administration is in progress. With effort, these concentrations can be reduced to 5 ppm in the operating room, and to 20 ppm in the dental operatory (see Chapter 6).

Concentrations reported in the recovery room are usually below levels reported for controlled operating room or dental anesthetizing locations, but definitive studies remain to be conducted.

REFERENCES

Allen, G.D., Goebel, W., Scaramella, J., et al. Apparatus to reduce trace nitrous oxide contamination in the dental operatory. *Anesth Prog.* November–December: 181–185, 1978.

Berner, O. Concentration and elimination of anaesthetic gases in operating theatres. *Acta Anaesthesiol Scand.* 22:46–54, 1978a.

_____. Concentration and elimination of anaesthetic gases in recovery rooms. *Acta Anaesthesiol Scand.* 22:55–57, 1978b.

Beynen, F.M., Knopp, T.J., and Rehder, K. Nitrous oxide exposure in the operating room. *Anesth Analg. (Cleve)* 57:216–223, 1978.

Bruce, D.L., and Linde, H.W. Halothane content in recovery room air. *Anesthesiology.* 36:517–518, 1972.

Campbell, R.L., Hannifan, M.A., Reist, P.C., et al. Exposure to anesthetic waste gas in oral surgery. *J Oral Surg.* 35:625–630, 1977.

Cleaton-Jones, P., Austin, J.C., Moyes, D.G., et al. Nitrous oxide contamination in dental surgeries using relative analgesia. *Br J Anaesth.* 50:1019–1024, 1978.

Cohen, E.N., Brown, B.W., Bruce, D.L., et al. Occupational disease among operating room personnel: A national study. *Anesthesiology.* 41:321–340, 1974.

Davenport, H.T., Halsey, M.J., Wardley-Smith, B., et al.

Measurement and reduction of occupational exposure to inhaled anaesthetics. *Br Med J.* 2:1219–1221, 1976.

Göthe, C.J., Ovrum, P., and Hallén, B. Exposure to anesthetic gases and ethanol during work in operating rooms. *Scand J Work Environ Health.* 2:96–106, 1976.

Hallén, B., Ehrner-Samuel, H., and Thomason, M. Measurements of halothane in the atmosphere of an operating theatre and in expired air and blood of the personnel during routine anaesthetic work. *Acta Anaesthesiol Scand.* 14:17–27, 1970.

Hannifan, M.A., Reist, P.C., and Campbell, R.L. Anesthetic waste gas exposure in dental surgery. *Am Ind Hyg Assoc J.* 39:69–73, 1978.

Kortilla, K., Pfäffli, P., and Ertama, P. Residual nitrous oxide in operating room personnel. *Acta Anaesthesiol Scand.* 22:635–639, 1978.

Linde, H.W., and Bruce, D.L. Occupational exposure of anesthetists to halothane, nitrous oxide, and radiation. *Anesthesiology.* 30:363–368, 1969.

Millard, R.J., and Corbett, T.H. Nitrous oxide concentrations in the dental operatory. *J Oral Surg.* 32:593–594, 1974.

Pfäffli, P., Nikki, P., and Ahlman, K. Halothane and nitrous oxide in end-tidal air and venous blood of surgical personnel. *Ann Clin Res.* 4:273–277, 1972.

Piziali, R.L., Whitcher, C., Sher, R., et al. Distribution of waste anesthetic gases in the operating room air. *Anesthesiology.* 45:487–494, 1976.

Scaramella, J., Allen, G.D., Adams, D., et al. Nitrous oxide pollution levels in oral surgery offices. *J Oral Surg.* 36:441–443, 1978.

Scheidt, M.J., Stanford, H.G., and Ayer, W.A. Measurement of waste gas contamination during nitrous oxide sedation in a non-ventilated dental operatory. *Anesth Prog.* March–April:38–42, 1977.

Swenson, R.D. Scavenging of dental anesthetic gases. *J Oral Surg.* 34:207–214, 1976.

Whitcher, C.E., Cohen, E.N., and Trudell, J.R. Chronic exposure to anesthetic gases in the operating room. *Anesthesiology.* 35:348–353, 1971.

Whitcher, C.E., Piziali, R., Sher, R., et al. *Development and Evaluation of Methods for the Elimination of Waste Anesthetic Gases and Vapors in Hospitals.* Washington, D.C.: U.S. Government Printing Office, 1975.

Whitcher, C.E., Zimmerman, D.C., Tonn, E.M., et al. Control of occupational exposure to nitrous oxide in the dental operatory. *J Am Dent Assoc.* 95:763–776, 1977.

3 Animal Experimental Studies

There is little doubt that prolonged administration of inhalation anesthesia results in both cellular and organ toxicity. Equally important to the development of this toxicity is the concentration of anesthetic employed. In most experimental studies, the inhalation anesthetic is administered in a clinical concentration for several hours, and the animal's postanesthetic recovery followed for only a brief period. By substituting a subclinical concentration of anesthetic, duration of the experiment may be significantly prolonged, and the animals successfully exposed for intervals extending to days or weeks. Although utilization of this subanesthetic concentration permits maintenance of viable fluid and caloric intake and allows long-term survival, it inevitably results in significant depression of a number of physiologic responses. Unfortunately, there are relatively few animal studies which have examined the more limited effects which follow exposure at trace-dose anesthetic concentration provided over very extensive periods of months to years. With trace-dose anesthetic concentrations, although measurable physiologic effects also occur, the associated toxicity is slow to develop, the responses are very subtle, and at times difficult to distinguish from control. Most important, under all circumstances of anesthetic exposure, toxicity depends upon the interrelated factors of length of exposure together with anesthetic concentration.

Acute toxic effects are sometimes associated with short-term clinical anesthetic administration. Primarily, these include reversible depression of the respiratory and circulatory systems. Long-term toxic effects following acute anesthetic administrations are relatively rare. When present, however, they are frequently irreversible and may involve significant damage to the liver, kidneys, and reproductive system.

Administration of anesthetics at subclinical concentration has the particular advantage of extended experimental exposure since the animal is able to maintain its own nutrition. Resultant long-term toxic effects, however, are generally similar to those effects which follow short-term clinical anesthetic administration, but additional responses also include decreases in body weight, hepatomegaly, splenomegaly, and disturbances in reproduction.

Long-term anesthetic exposure at trace-anesthetic concentrations (10 to 1000 ppm) is difficult to accomplish in the laboratory. Specially designed exposure chambers are required, and large numbers of animals are needed for statistical validity. The toxic responses which do occur are usually at or below the threshold level and are frequently difficult to define. Responses also vary significantly with the experimental species. While the adverse toxic effects which ultimately appear may be similar to those which follow short-term clinical or subclinical exposure, they differ in that the long-term, low-dose response additionally involves exposure to by-products of anesthetic metabolism whose formation has been accentuated through an accompanying induction of liver drug-metabolizing enzyme systems.

Present widespread interest in investigations of animal toxicity at trace anesthetic levels reflects our growing concern with the similar exposure that occurs clinically in the operating room and dental operatory. Unfortunately, calculation of the involved population indicates that large numbers of health professionals are occupationally exposed to the long-term effects of waste anesthetic gases in the course of their medical or dental employment. It has been estimated by the National Institute of Occupational Safety and Health (NIOSH) that a minimum of 214,000 workers in the United States, including anesthesiologists, nurse anesthetists, operating room nurses and technicians, oral surgeons, dentists and their assistants, and veterinarians and their assistants, are potentially exposed to waste anesthetic gases (Geraci, 1977).

Considering the inherent difficulties involved in conducting human studies of this type, it becomes especially important to develop an experimental animal model to study the potential health hazard. Since any animal studies equivalent to the long-term human exposure must extend for many months, experiments necessarily involve a significant portion of an animal's lifespan. Such experiments are arduous and costly, and the measurable incidence of resultant toxic responses is low. Interspecies differences and required correlations of these animal data to humans offer additional difficulties. Unfortunately, despite considerable effort, data obtained thus far in a large number of experimental species show only limited correlation to the human epidemiologic studies. The problems are significant.

EXPOSURE STUDIES AT SUBANESTHETIC CONCENTRATION

Although our major clinical concern relates to long-term exposure occurring at trace-anesthetic concentration, data obtained in experiments which have been conducted at higher subclinical concentration are useful. In an early study, Chenoweth et al. (1972) examined comparative chronic inhalation toxicities of methoxyflurane, halothane, and diethyl ether in several animal species (rats, guinea pigs, and rabbits). The anesthetics were administered at approximately one-tenth their clinically used concentration. Anesthetic exposures took place in large exposure chambers for several hours per day, five days per week, throughout a period of seven weeks. At the time of sacrifice, the authors noted a significant decrease in body weight in several species following exposure to both halothane and methoxyflurane. Most significant were the increases noted in the liver-to-body-weight ratio. Changes in SGOT and SGPT were limited to methoxyflurane, although a number of animals evidenced focal hepatic infiltration following either halothane or methoxyflurane administration. Of particular interest, diethyl ether showed no hepatotoxic response, leading the authors to conclude that metabolites from ether may be less toxic than those derived from the halogenated anesthetics. The authors further suggested that these observed results may bear an association to the question of chronic toxicity in anesthetic-exposed operating room personnel.

Stevens et al. (1975) conducted chronic exposure studies in mice, rats, and guinea pigs at both subanesthetic and trace-concentration ranges. Exposures were continuous for five weeks and included administrations of halothane, isoflurane, or diethyl ether during the phase of rapid body growth. Halothane produced the greatest decrement in weight gain and increase in hepatic degeneration. The changes with isoflurane or diethyl ether were relatively small (Figures 3-1 and 3-2). Although there were significant interspecies differences (guinea pigs proved to be the most susceptible species), livers from the halothane-treated animals demonstrated degenerative changes which increased in frequency as exposures increased from 15 to 300 ppm. This dose-response relationship suggested to the authors that halothane acted as a hepatotoxin in the classic sense. The data further indicated that metabolism of halothane might be a significant factor in its toxicity, since isoflurane evidenced low toxicity and is significantly less metabolized than is halothane. Ether proved essentially innocuous. Although the possibility of occult liver injury exists, the present findings cannot be directly applied to those trace-anesthetic levels associated with operating room exposure. In Stevens' studies, liver damage was present only at levels of halothane 10 to 15 times the concentration found in the immediate area of the anesthesia machine.

Kripke et al. (1976) investigated the effects of chronic exposure to subanesthetic concentrations of nitrous oxide with respect to spermatogenesis in the male rat. The animals were exposed intermittently to 20% nitrous oxide, 20% oxygen, and 60% nitrogen for a maximum of 35 days. Evidence of injury to the seminiferous tubules was present in some animals by the second day, and by the fourteenth day,

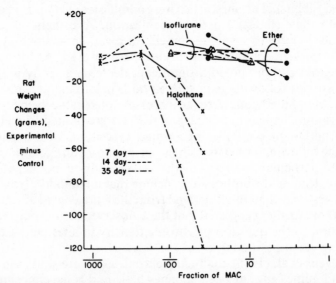

Figure 3-1 Body weight changes in anesthetic-exposed rats in relation to type of anesthetic, dose, and duration of exposure. (From Stevens et al., *Anesthesiology.* 42:408–419, 1975. Reprinted by permission of the publisher, J.B. Lippincott, and the author.)

testicular damage was noted in all animals. Toxic effects from the anesthetic appeared to be confined to the spermatogenic cells, with reductions in the number of mature spermatozoa and the appearance of multinucleated forms. Damage in the spermatogonial cells was mirrored by changes in testicular weights, which significantly decreased during and immediately following nitrous oxide exposure (Figure 3-3). Recovery of normal spermatogenesis, however, occurred within 3 days of the animals' return to room air, and testicular weights also returned toward normal values within 6 days of rebreathing room air. Serum testosterone levels were not significantly affected during the prolonged subanesthetic exposures. Although dose-response levels were not provided, the testicular damage present after exposure to an even higher nitrous oxide concentration (40%) appeared to be accelerated in both time and severity. Again, although these studies are of significant interest, their implications to the clinical operating room situation must be carefully evaluated in terms of the very high nitrous oxide concentration employed, i.e., 200,000 ppm.

Lansdown et al. (1976) examined the effects of maternal exposure to subanesthetic concentrations of halothane upon fetal development. Pregnant Sprague-Dawley rats were exposed to halothane for eight hours daily during days 8 through 12 of gestation at concentrations of

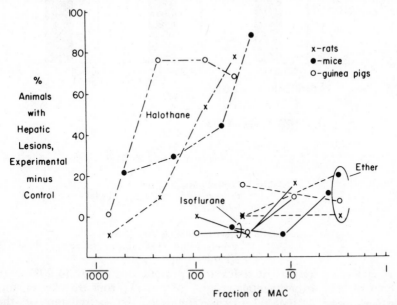

Figure 3-2 Incidence of hepatic degenerative lesions in mice, rats, and guinea pigs after 35-day exposures to various doses of halothane, isoflurane, and diethyl ether. (From Stevens et al., *Anesthesiology*. 42:408–419, 1975. Reprinted by permission of the publisher, J.B. Lippincott, and the author.)

anesthetic in air varying from 50 to 3200 ppm. Special care was taken during this period to avoid the effects of experimental stress by putting the breeding cages directly into the exposure chamber. Fetal growth was affected only at the highest halothane concentrations, i.e., in excess of 1600 ppm. Fetal anomalies were infrequent and did not appear to be exposure related. The authors concluded that exposure of the pregnant animals to these subanesthetic concentrations of halothane exerted no appreciable effect on fetal development.

Later studies by Pope, Halsey, and Lansdown (1978) investigated comparative fetotoxicity in rats following chronic exposures to

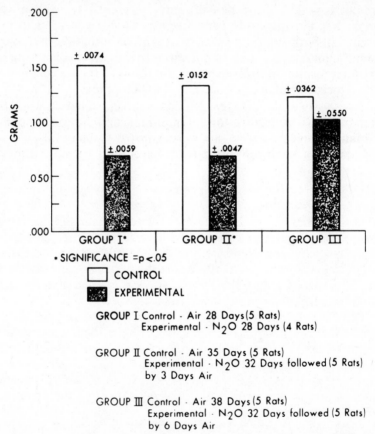

Figure 3-3 Dry weights of testes after prolonged exposure to 20% N_2O in control and experimental groups of rats. (From Kripke et al., *Anesthesiology.* 44:104–113, 1976. Reprinted by permission of the publisher, J.B. Lippincott, and the author.)

halothane, nitrous oxide, or methoxyflurane. In their rat model system, the animals were exposed to high subanesthetic concentrations eight hours per day throughout the 21-day gestation period. Although fetal growth retardation occurred with all anesthetics at the higher levels, this was unaccompanied by significant fetal loss, and there were no changes in the number of implantations per litter.

An extensive study of fertility, reproduction, and postnatal survival in mice chronically exposed to subanesthetic concentrations of halothane was carried out by Wharton et al. (1978). Male and female mice were treated five or seven days per week for nine-week periods prior to mating, and exposure continued throughout pregnancy. Halothane exposures ranged from 0.025 to 4.0 MAC (minimum alveolar concentration) hours per day. No adverse effects on reproduction were observed at levels below 0.1 MAC hour, but higher exposure levels were associated with decreased fetal length and decreased weight gains. Pregnancy rate, implantation rate, and number of live fetuses per litter were also significantly decreased at a level of 1.2 MAC hours per day. Subsequent matings of unexposed females to halothane-exposed males resulted in normal reproductive performance. This result suggests that the adverse reproductive changes observed when both males and females were exposed are greater in females. Results of this study additionally serve to define a threshold level of halothane exposure at which reproductive toxicity occurs in this species.

In combination, most of the preceding studies suggest that reproductive effects are associated with long-term anesthetic exposure at subanesthetic concentration. Although the effects appear dose related, one must consider that serious toxicity was only observed at concentrations of anesthetic 10 to 100 times greater than those normally present in an unscavenged operating room.

Only limited data are available which define the carcinogenic potential of anesthetics administered at subanesthetic concentration. Although hepatic malignancy in the rat has been reported following high-dose oral administrations of both chloroform and trichloroethylene (Eschenbrenner, 1945; Saffioti, 1975), recent exposure studies in mice with enflurane, isoflurane, halothane, methoxyflurane, and nitrous oxide at levels ranging from 1/32 to 1/2 MAC have proven negative (Eger et al., 1978). It would appear that projections of results obtained at subanesthetic concentrations to effects associated with trace levels of anesthetic in the operating room, while useful, carry significant hazard in interpretation, even when problems of species variation are disregarded.

EXPOSURE STUDIES AT TRACE ANESTHETIC CONCENTRATION

One of the first experimental studies evaluating animal exposure to trace anesthetic concentrations (halothane 16 ppm) was reported by Bruce (1973). In this study, several strains of mice were exposed intermittently to air or to halothane in air for seven hours daily, 5 days per week, for periods of six weeks, and then mated. The mice were sacrificed 18 days later. Exposed pregnant animals showed no significant changes in fertility or in fetal resorption rate compared to control. Splenic weights in male mice were within normal range except for a slight decrease in splenic weight in one of the SWR strains. There were no other differences noted between various strains.

Studies conducted that same year with a different experimental species and another anesthetic, nitrous oxide, produced differing results. Corbett et al. (1973) exposed pregnant rats to varying concentrations of nitrous oxide for 8- to 24-hour periods during selected days of gestation. The number of implantations per rat in animals exposed for 24 hours was significantly reduced following exposures to both 1000 and 15,000 ppm nitrous oxide concentrations compared to control. Exposure effects were noted in a dose-dependent fashion, and animals exposed to only 100 ppm nitrous oxide for 8 hours showed no reduction in the number of implantations. Although a published report is not available, Ferstandig (1978) reported that a repeat study of nitrous oxide exposure by these same authors proved negative.

Toxic anesthetic effects, however, have been reported in rat embryo and fetal development following exposure to trace concentrations of chloroform anesthesia. Schwetz, Leong, and Gehring (1974) exposed pregnant Sprague-Dawley rats to from 30 to 300 ppm chloroform for seven hours per day on the sixth through fifteenth days of gestation. Exposure to chloroform caused an apparent decrease in the conception rate and a high incidence of fetal resorption, retarded fetal development, and decreased fetal body measurements (Table 3-1). Chloroform, while not highly teratogenic, was markedly embryotoxic.

Production of an enduring learning deficit was demonstrated by Quimby et al. (1974a) in rats exposed to 10 ppm halothane from day 1 of conception through the sixtieth day of age. When tested as to their abilities to learn two maze tasks, the exposed animals made approximately 30% more errors than did the control group (Figure 3-4). Animals exposed only during three months of their adult life did not show a significantly different response from control. These data suggest that the critical exposure period with respect to anesthetics is

Table 3-1
Effect of Chloroform Inhalation in Pregnant Rats Upon Fetal Resorption and Development

	Air	30 ppm	Chloroform 100 ppm	300 ppm
Percent pregnancies	77	71	82	15*
Percent resorptions	8	8	6	61*
Sex ratio (M:F)	53:47	53:47	55:45	34:66*
Fetal body weight (g)	5.59 ± 0.36	5.51 ± 0.20	5.59 ± 0.24	3.42 ± 0.02*
Fetal crown-rump length (mm)	43.5 ± 1.1	42.5 ± 0.6*	43.6 ± 0.7	36.9 ± 0.2*

Source: Schwetz, Leong, and Gehring, *Toxicol Appl Pharmacol.* 28:442–451, 1974. Reprinted by permission of the publisher, Academic Press, Inc., and the authors.
*p < 0.05 compared to control.

limited to early fetal development. Significant learning disabilities result in the rat following exposure to levels of halothane comparable to those trace concentrations present in unscavenged operating rooms. Correlative to the behavioral deficits noted, tissue samples obtained from the superior parasagittal cerebral cortex of exposed animals indicated electron microscopic evidence of neural degeneration and failure in formation of the synaptic web in 30% of postsynaptic membranes. A later study by Quimby, Katz, and Bowman (1975) analyzed rates of learning for halothane-exposed and halothane-unexposed rats. The authors reported that animals exposed to this anesthetic during early development made 30% more errors than the control group when tested by shock-motivated and food-motivated discrimination tasks. The relative rates of learning, however, were similar for both groups.

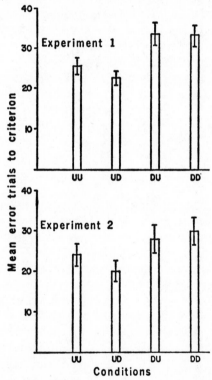

Figure 3-4 Errors in learning as a function of conditions of exposure to halothane. The UU group was unexposed; the UD group was exposed from day 60 of age on; the DU group was exposed from conception on; the DD group exposed during both periods. (From Quimby et al., *Science.* 185:625–627, 1974a. Reprinted by permission of the publisher and of the author.)

Chang et al. (1974) subsequently reported ultrastructural changes in the central nervous system following chronic exposure of young adult rats to trace levels of halothane (10 ppm). Following eight weeks of exposure, collapse of the neuronal rough endoplasmic reticulum was observed, with dilatation of the Golgi complex and focal cytoplasmic vacuolation within many cortical neurons. After exposure to 500 ppm halothane, there was more severe dilatation and vacuolar degeneration of the Golgi complex. Membraneous degeneration of the neuronal mitochondria, intracellular edema of the glial cells, and necrosis of the cortical neurons were also found. These findings suggest that halothane may behave as a neurotoxin in both the neonatal and adult nervous systems.

Over the next two years, Chang and associates published a series of five papers reporting ultrastructural changes in liver, kidney, and nervous tissues in rats exposed to 10 ppm halothane for eight hours per day, six days per week, or to 500 ppm for four weeks. These results are summarized in an overview by Chang and Katz (1976). Renal lesions were found centered in the proximal convoluted tubules with degeneration of mitochondria and accumulation and fusion of lysosomes. Brain degenerative changes included severe vacuolation of the Golgi complex, collapse of the rough endoplasmic reticulum, and focal disruption of the neuronal nuclear membrane. Hepatic damage included degenerative changes in the mitochondria and endoplasmic reticulum, and in bile canaliculi. These ultrastructural studies, however, have proved difficult to evaluate since adequate quantification was not supplied, and control data are not available. Nonetheless, the extensive pathologic changes reported to be associated with exposure to only 10 ppm halothane are remarkable.

A most significant series of long-term, low-level anesthetic exposure experiments have recently been reported from the Hazelton Laboratories by Coate, Kapp, and Lewis (1979). These investigators exposed adult male and female rats for 60 days prior to mating to either 1 and 50 ppm or to 10 and 500 ppm of halothane with nitrous oxide, respectively, for seven hours per day, five days per week. Inseminated females were then exposed on either days 1 through 15 or days 6 through 15, and their pups evaluated for teratologic effects. The former group of exposed animals were allowed to deliver normally, and the latter were delivered by Caesarean section on day 10. Males were exposed for an additional 40 weeks, after which cytogenetic studies were undertaken of bone marrow and spermatogonial cells.

Among the naturally delivered females, the mean number of corpora lutea was reduced in both exposure groups compared to control (Table 3-2). The number of implantations was reduced in those animals exposed to the higher anesthetic concentration, their

Table 3-2
**Group Mean Ovarian and Uterine Data for Reproductive Indicies
and Litter Data for Mated Female Rats Exposed during Days 1
through 15 of Gestation and Delivered Normally**

	Control	Low Exposure*	High Exposure†
Ovarian corpora lutea	19.5 ± 3.8	15.4 ± 5.9‡	13.2 ± 5.2‡
Uterine implantation sites	10.9 ± 5.5	7.5 ± 6.2	3.8 ± 6.2‡
Implantation efficiency (%)	56	49	29
Postimplantation loss index (%)	14	15	28
Gestation index (%)	94	92	57

Source: Coate, Kapp, and Lewis, *Anesthesiology,* 50:310–318, 1979.
Reprinted by permission of the publisher, J.B. Lippincott, and the authors.

*Exposed to halothane 1 ppm and N_2O 50 ppm.
†Exposed to halothane 10 ppm and N_2O 500 ppm.
‡p 0.05 exposed versus control.

postimplantation loss index was increased, and the gestation index reduced.

Females exposed during day 6 through 16 of gestation and delivered by Caesarean section showed a reduced level of response, with significant decreases noted only in fetal weight and fetal length. No teratologic effects and no abortifacient effects were observed following exposure of pregnant females during organogenesis, nor were they associated with prior exposure of the males.

On the other hand, significant cytogenetic damage to chromosomes in bone marrow cells and in spermatogonial cells was found in the long-term exposed male rats at both levels of chronic exposure compared to their control (Table 3-3). Aberrations noted included marker chromosomes (exchange figures, rings, and miscellaneous markers), but excluded gaps. There appeared to be a dose-related effect with respect to the percent of animals with aberrant chromosomes and the mean number of cells showing aberrations.

The results of these studies strongly suggest that chronic exposure to very low levels of halothane combined with nitrous oxide in a proportion similar to that used in surgical anesthesia may produce adverse effects on the reproductive process and on male chromosomes in vivo. Although the study findings were significant at two dose levels, the experiments did not address the question of whether nitrous oxide or halothane alone could produce the observed effects, nor did they consider other possible concomitant influences such as stress, etc. Nonetheless, the implications of these results to low-level operating room anesthetic exposure are serious.

Coate, Ulland, and Lewis (1979) investigated the effect of low-level, halothane-nitrous oxide exposure on carcinogenesis in the rat. Three groups of 50 male and female Fischer-344 rats were exposed to air, to halothane 1 ppm and nitrous oxide 50 ppm, or to halothane 10 ppm and nitrous oxide 500 ppm seven hours per day, five days per week, for 104 weeks. No evidence was found for exposure-related effects on body weight, appearance, behavior, or survival rates.

Table 3-3
Numbers of Animals and Incidence of Bone Marrow and Spermatogonial Cells Showing Aberrations in Chromosomal Structure

Condition	No. Animals	Animals with Aberrant Cells (%)	Cells with Aberrations (%)
Bone marrow			
Control	38	28.9(11)	1.6(15)
Low exposure*	37	59.5(22)‡	3.2(30)§
High exposure†	38	68.4(26)‡	5.3(50)‡
Spermatogonia			
Control	35	48.5(17)	2.6(23)
Low exposure	35	77.1(27)§	6.7(59)‡
High exposure	30	86.7(26)‡	12.6(95)‡

Source: Coate, Kapp, and Lewis, *Anesthesiology,* 50:310–318, 1979. Reprinted by permission of the publisher, J.B. Lippincott, and the authors.
*Exposed to halothane 1 ppm and N_2O 50 ppm.
†Exposed to halothane 10 ppm and N_2O 500 ppm.
‡$p < 0.01$ exposed versus control.
§$p < 0.05$ exposed versus control.
( )indicates number of animals with aberrant cells or number of cells with aberrations.

Histopathologic evaluation of major organs and of the reticuloen-dothelial system revealed no enhancement of the spontaneous tumor rate nor any unusual neoplasms. Although the experimental design did not permit detection of small increases in the incidence of neoplastic disease, there was no suggestion of significant tumorigenic effect. Despite the lack of positive results in these experiments, one should keep in mind the difficulties in interpreting cancer data obtained from animal studies that employ small populations. In addition, these studies must be evaluated in terms of the significant problems involved in attempting to compare effects produced at high-dose,[1] clinical-dose, subanesthetic-dose, or trace-dose levels of anesthetic.

Although the number of animal experimental studies conducted at trace-dose levels of anesthetic is limited and the results variable, it appears that evidence for a significant number of physiologic altera-tions exists. Fetotoxicity in the animal appears to have its counterpart in humans, but relative susceptibilities are indeterminate. Data on chromosomal aberration in the rat are highly suggestive, but no equivalent information exists in humans. Data on the susceptibility to cancer in animals at trace anesthetic dose exposure have thus far proven negative.

REFERENCES

Bruce, D.L. Murine fertility unaffected by traces of halothane. *Anesthesiology.* 38:473–477, 1973.

Chang, L.W., Dudley, A.W., Lee, Y.K., et al. Ultrastructural changes in the nervous system after chronic exposure to halothane. *Exp Neurol.* 45:209–219, 1974.

Chang, L.W., and Katz, J. Pathologic effects of chronic halothane inhalation: An overview. *Anesthesiology.* 45:640–653, 1976.

Chenoweth, M.B., Leong, B.K.J., Sparschu, G.L., et al. Tox-icities of methoxyflurane, halothane, and diethyl ether in laboratory animals in repeated inhalation at subanesthetic concentrations. Edited by B.R. Fink. In *Cellular Biology and Toxicity of Anesthetics.* Baltimore, Maryland: Williams and Wilkins Company, 1972.

Coate, W.B., Kapp, R.W., and Lewis, T.R. Chronic low-level halothane-nitrous oxide exposure: Reproductive and cytogenetic effects in rats. *Anesthesiology.* 50:310–318, 1979.

Coate, W.B., Ulland, B.M., and Lewis, T.R. Chronic low-level

---

[1]National Cancer Institute studies indicate induction of hepatic malignancy in rats following their ingestion of large oral doses of chloroform or trichloroethylene (Eschenbrenner, *J Natl Cancer Inst.* 5:251–255, 1945; Saffioti, *J Natl Cancer Inst.* Memorandum Alert, March 21, 1975).

halothane-nitrous oxide exposure: Lack of carcinogenic effect in rats. *Anesthesiology.* 50:306–309, 1979.

Corbett, T.H., Cornell, R.G., Endres, J.L., et al. Effects of low concentrations of nitrous oxide on rat pregnancy. *Anesthesiology.* 39:299–301, 1973.

Eger, E.I., White, A.E., Brown, C.L., et al. A test of the carcinogenicity of enflurane, isoflurane, methoxyflurane, and nitrous oxide in mice. *Anesth Analg (Cleve).* 57:678–694, 1978.

Eschenbrenner, A.B. Induction of hematomas in mice by repeated oral administration of chloroform with observations on sex differences. *J Natl Cancer Inst.* 5:251–255, 1945.

Ferstandig, L.L. Trace concentration of anesthetic gases: A critical review of their disease potential. *Anesth Analg (Cleve).* 57:328–345, 1978.

Geraci, C.L. Operating room pollution: Governmental perspectives and guidelines. *Anesth Analg (Cleve).* 56:775–777, 1977.

Kripke, B.J., Kelman, A.D., Shah, K., et al. Testicular reaction to prolonged exposure to nitrous oxide. *Anesthesiology.* 44:104–113, 1976.

Lansdown, A.B.G., Pope, W.D.B., Halsey, M.J., et al. Analysis of fetal development in rats following maternal exposure to subanesthetic concentrations of halothane. *Teratology.* 13:229–304, 1976.

Pope, W.D.B., Halsey, M.J., and Lansdown, A.B.G. Fetotoxicity in rats following chronic exposure to halothane, nitrous oxide, or methoxyflurane. *Anesthesiology.* 48:11–16, 1978.

Quimby, K.L., Aschkenase, L.J., Bowman, R.E., et al. Enduring learning deficits and cerebral synaptic malformation from exposure to 10 parts of halothane per million. *Science.* 185:625–627, 1974a.

Quimby, K.L., Katz, J., and Bowman, R.E. Behavioral consequences in rats from chronic exposure to 10 ppm halothane during early development. *Anesth Analg (Cleve).* 54:628–633, 1975b.

Saffioti, U. Memorandum alert. *J Natl Cancer Inst.* March 21, 1975.

Schwetz, B.A., Leong, B.K.J., and Gehring, P.J. Embryo- and fetotoxicity of inhaled chloroform in rats. *Toxicol Appl Pharmacol.* 28:442–451, 1974.

Stevens, W.C., Eger, E.I., White, A., et al. Comparative toxicities of halothane, isoflurane, and diethyl ether at subanesthetic concentrations in laboratory animals. *Anesthesiology.* 42:408–419, 1975.

Wharton, R.S., Mazze, R.I., Baden, J.M., et al. Fertility, reproduction, and postnatal survival in mice chronically exposed to halothane. *Anesthesiology.* 48:167–174, 1978.

4 The Human Health Hazard

EPIDEMIOLOGIC STUDIES

Probably the first epidemiologic study designed to survey occupational health hazards in anesthetists was that conducted by Vaisman (1967). In this study, Vaisman distributed questionnaires to 354 fellow Russian anesthetists who constituted approximately 15% of the active specialty and included 110 women. The major purpose of the investigation was to examine working conditions of Russian anesthetists, which she had reason to believe were seriously inadequate. The results of the survey indicated a high incidence of minor health complaints among anesthetists, including headache (78%), fatigue (85%), and pruritus (87%). These complaints were found to be associated with inadequate ventilation, defective anesthesia equipment, and poor operating room architectural design. Additionally, many of the anesthetists ascribed their health problems to excessive work loads and long, continuous hours spent in the operating theater.

Unfortunately, Vaisman's study design had a significant deficiency in that it lacked the necessary control population. In the absence of such control, it was tempting to dismiss her reported findings as vague polysymptomatology. What generated attention, however, was the unexpected observation that of 31 pregnancies recorded among the 110 female anesthetists, 18 terminated in spontaneous abortion. Only 7 pregnancies in the overall group were considered normal.

Although Vaisman's original intent was to survey anesthetic working conditions, her startling findings served to focus broad attention upon the previously unsuspected question of obstetrical problems among female anesthetists, including possible increases in spontaneous miscarriage rate and in congenital abnormalities in their children.

As a result of this initial report, two additional small surveys were subsequently initiated. Askrog and Harvald (1970) reported a survey of 578 nurses and 174 male and female anesthetists working in Danish anesthesia departments. These authors analyzed a total of 604 pregnancies, of which 212 occurred prior to employment, and 392 took place subsequent to the women's work in the anesthesia department. The spontaneous abortion rate proved to be significantly higher in those women pregnant during employment compared to those pregnant before employment (Table 4-1). Although this difference was statistically significant, this study was deficient in that the analysis did not allow for the increased number of miscarriages to be anticipated associated with increasing age of the mother during the four-year period of study. A rather surprising result in this study was the unanticipated finding that wives of male anesthetists also experienced an increased spontaneous miscarriage rate, implying an indirect obstetrical effect in women who themselves had had no direct exposure to the operating room environment.

The following year, Cohen, Bellville, and Brown (1971) examined the incidence of spontaneous miscarriage in a series of operating room nurses and physician anesthetists in the state of California and compared these women to working nurses and physicians not employed in the operating room. Each nurse was personally interviewed by a nurse-psychologist team, and the physicians were asked to respond to a mail questionnaire. Since the study design did not permit exact determination of the influence of duration of operating room exposure upon subsequent pregnancy, exposure to the operating room arbitrarily assigned the respondent to the experimental group. Sixty-seven operating room nurses reported a 29.7% spontaneous miscarriage rate compared to an 8.8% control rate in the general duty nurses. The incidence of spontaneous miscarriage was noted to be even higher in female anesthesiologists (37.8%), and the control

Table 4-1
Rate of Spontaneous Miscarriages before and after Employment in the Anesthesia Department

	No. Live Births	No. Miscarriages	Miscarriages/ Pregnancies (%)
Anesthetic nurses			
Before employment	75	10	11.8
After employment	191	38	16.6
Female anesthetists			
Before employment	8	0	–
After employment	19	7	26.9
Wives of male anesthetists			
Before employment	110	9	8.2
After employment	110	28	20.3

Source: Askrog and Harvald, *Nord Med.* 83:498–504, 1970. Reprinted by permission of the author.

group of nonoperating room female physicians demonstrated an incidence of spontaneous miscarriage similar to that of the nonoperating room nurse control group (Table 4-2). Miscarriages were noted to occur earlier in both operating room nurses and physician anesthetists compared to their control groups (eight versus tenth week), suggesting a possible fetal lethality associated with operating room exposure.

A larger epidemiologic survey was conducted in Great Britain (Knill-Jones et al., 1972). This study examined 563 female anesthetists who were in turn compared to a group of 828 nonanesthetist physicians taken from the *Medical Register.* Reply rates of 82% and 80% were achieved for anesthetists and controls, respectively. Results of this survey (Table 4-3) confirmed the presence of a significantly higher miscarriage rate (18.2%) for anesthetists working during pregnancy compared to their control group (14.7%), but not when compared to nonworking anesthetists (13.7%). Anesthetists who worked during pregnancy also produced a significantly higher percentage of children with congenital abnormalities (6.5%) compared to mothers not at work during the first or second trimester of their pregnancy (2.5%),

Table 4-2
Rate of Spontaneous Miscarriages in Operating Room-Exposed
Nurses and Physicians Compared to Control

	No. Respondents	No. Live Births	No. Miscarriages	Miscarriages/Pregnancies (%)
General duty nurses	92	31	3	8.6
O.R. nurses	67	26	10	29.7*
General duty personnel	81	52	6	10.3
Physician anesthetists	50	33	14	37.8†

Source: Cohen, Bellville, and Brown. *Anesthesiology* 35:343–347, 1971. Reprinted by permission of the publisher, J.B. Lippincott, and of the author.
*p < 0.05 compared to control.
†p < 0.01 compared to control.

Table 4-3
Rate of Spontaneous Miscarriages and of Congenital Anomalies among Children of Female Anesthetists at Work during Pregnancy, Female Anesthetists Not at Work during Pregnancy, and a Control Group.

	No. Respondents	No. Live Births	No. Miscarriages	No. Congenital Anomalies	Miscarriages/ Pregnancies (%)	Live Births/ Congenital Anomalies (%)
Anesthetists	563					
Not at work		290	46	7	13.7	2.5
At work		603	134	39	18.2*	6.5†
Control physicians	828	1835	315	89	14.0	4.9

Source: Knill-Jones et al., *Lancet* 2:1326–1328, 1972. Tables 4-3, 4-14, and 4-15 reprinted by permission of the publisher and of the author.

*p < 0.025 anesthetists at work compared to control physicians.
†p < 0.02 anesthetist at work compared to those not at work.

but did not differ from control (4.9%). Involuntary infertility among the 563 anesthetists was found to be 12%, a rate significantly different from that of the control physician group (6%).

A small-scale study conducted in Finland by Rosenberg and Kirves (1973) suggested an alternative explanation for the higher miscarriage rates noted among operating room staff. These authors interviewed 300 Finnish women working as anesthesia, scrub, casualty, and intensive-care nurses with regard to the fate of their pregnancies (Table 4-4). Among 124 scrub nurses, the incidence of spontaneous abortion was found to be 21.5% during employment; among 43 intensive-care nurses, 16.7%; among 58 anesthesia nurses, 15.0%; and among 75 casualty nurses, 8.3%. It was further observed that scrub nurses and intensive-care nurses had earlier miscarriages (9.3 weeks and 10.4 weeks, respectively) compared to the anesthesia nurses (11.1) weeks. On this basis, the authors suggested that the higher incidence and earlier miscarriages among scrub and intensive-care nurses compared to anesthesia nurses might be reasonably accounted for by the greater stress and longer working hours required of the former women. However, statistical analysis of the data did not reveal significant differences between either of these groups compared to anesthesia nurses. On the other hand, when the authors grouped together women who worked in the operating room (anesthesia nurses plus scrub nurses) and compared these women to nonoperating-room-employed nurses (casuality nurses plus intensive-care nurses), there was a statistically significant increase in the spontaneous miscarriage rate for operating room-exposed nurses (19.5%) compared to nurses not exposed to the operating room (11.4%).

Corbett et al. (1973b) conducted a survey designed to answer questions regarding a possible increase in cancer among operating room-exposed personnel. Among 621 female nurse anesthetists in Michigan participating in this survey, 33 respondents to the questionnaire indicated the presence of malignancy. The age-adjusted incidence of cancer was 1333/100,000 in nurse anesthetists compared to only 403/100,000 reported in a comparable age group taken from the *Connecticut Tumor Registry*. This threefold increase in cancer was found to be statistically significant, although only when applied to analysis of the seven cases of cancer occurring during the single year 1971.

The following year, an extensive survey of occupational disease among operating room personnel was undertaken by the American Society of Anesthesiologists (ASA) Ad Hoc Committee in cooperation with NIOSH (Cohen et al., 1974). This national survey involved

Table 4-4
Rate of Sponteneous Miscarriages During Employment
for Four Different Nursing Groups

	No. Respondents	No. Pregnancies	No. Miscarriages	Miscarriages/Pregnancies (%)	
Anesthesia nurses	58	80	12	15.0 ⎫	19.5*
Scrub nurses	124	177	37	21.5 ⎭	
Casualty nurses	75	96	8	8.3 ⎫	11.4
Intensive-care nurses	43	54	9	16.7 ⎭	

Source: Rosenberg and Kirves, *Acta Anaesth Scand.* 53:37–42, 1973. Reprinted by permission of the publisher, Munksgaard International Publishers.
*$p < 0.05$ operating room-employed nurses compared to nonoperating room-employed nurses.

the mailing of questionnaires to 49,585 exposed operating room personnel in three professional societies—ASA, AANA (American Association of Nurse Anesthetists), AORN/T (Association of Operating Room Nurses/Association of Operating Room Technicians)—as well as to 23,911 operating room-unexposed individuals in two professional societies serving as a comparison group—AAP (American Association of Pediatrics) and ANA (American Nursing Association). The former professional groups represented essentially all personnel in the United States potentially exposed to trace gases in the operating room environment. Usable responses were obtained from 40,044 individuals, representing a return rate varying from a high of 75.5% among female members of the ASA to a low of 41.8% among female members of the ANA.[1]

Analysis of these results indicated that female anesthesiologists, nurse anesthetists, and operating room nurses and technicians exposed to the operating room during their first trimester of pregnancy, as well as during the preceding year, were subject to a statistically significant increased risk of spontaneous abortion—1.3 to 2 times that of the unexposed nonoperating room personnel (Table 4-5). Certain difficulties were present in making direct comparison between members of the different professional societies. Pediatricians and physician anesthetists, as well as nurse anesthetists, operating room nurses, and general duty nurses, have different professional training and do not represent the same populations and therefore might respond differently to the questionnaire. This problem of intergroup comparison was partially circumvented by employing intragroup comparisons using members of the same professional society. When women within a single professional society were separated into a group exposed to the operating room during their first trimester and one year preceding pregnancy, and compared to a second group of women in the same society who were not so exposed, results were remarkably similar to those found in the intergroup comparison.

Although each group of women working in the operating room experienced a spontaneous miscarriage rate higher than that of women outside the operating room, there was no evidence to indicate an earlier abortion rate for these individuals, nor was there any decrease in the sex ratio of live-born babies. The spontaneous abor-

---

[1]The low response rates found in the two control groups (AAP and AANA) were of serious concern. In an attempt to determine if the nonresponding group was in any way different from those who returned their questionnaires, a third mailing was sent to the remaining female members of the AAP. This additional mailing increased the total return rate for female members of the AAP group to 72.1%. Comparative analysis of returns from the three mailings indicated no significant differences in responses to the three mailings.

Table 4-5
Spontaneous Miscarriage Rates for Female Respondents
All data adjusted for age and smoking habit. Rates are per 100
pregnancies (excluding therapeutic abortions).

Organization	Rate	Organization	Rate	p
ASA	17.1 ± 2.0 (468)	AAP	8.9 ± 1.8 (308)	< 0.01
AANA	17.0 ± 0.9 (1826)	ANA	15.1 ± 0.9 (1948)	0.07
AORN/T	19.5 ± 0.9 (2781)	ANA	15.1 ± 0.9 (1948)	< 0.01

Source: Cohen et al., *Anesthesiology* 41:321–340, 1974, Tables 4-5
through 4-11 reprinted by permission of the publisher, J.B.
Lippincott, and of the author.

tion rate reported in wives of male respondents, when standardized
for age and smoking habit of the spouse, provided no evidence that
male exposure to the operating room resulted in an increased number
of abortions.

There was, however, evidence for an increased risk of congenital
abnormalities among live-born children of female anesthesiologists
(5.9%) compared to children of unexposed female pediatricians
(3.0%). Among female nurse anesthetists, the abnormality rate was
9.6% compared to 7.6% in general duty nurses (Table 4-6). As with
spontaneous miscarriage rates, intergroup analysis of congenital abnormality rates between different professional societies introduced
difficulties in making direct comparisons.[2] An intragroup comparison
among members of the same society which contrasted women exposed
to the operating room with unexposed women resulted in congenital
abnormality rates similar to those obtained by the intergroup
comparisons.

Of considerable interest, a statistically significant increase in the
incidence of congenital abnormalities was also noted among children

[2]It appears that nurses and nurse technicians have a different reporting rate
for congenital abnormalities (and spontaneous miscarriages) than do physicians. These differences are likely dependent upon both work experience and
educational background. Data received were analyzed as reported on the
questionnaire without further opportunity to determine their accuracy.

58

of the wives of operating room-exposed physician anesthetists (Table 4-7). This unanticipated increase in congenital abnormalities present in children of women unexposed to the operating room is of particular concern and suggests a defect transmitted through the male. Unfortunately, the limited number of male nurse respondents prevented similar analysis of the data with respect to their wives.

Table 4-6
Congenital Abnormality Rates (Excluding Skin) for Children of Female Respondents
All data adjusted for age and smoking habit. Rates are per 100 live births.

Organization	Rate	Organization	Rate	p
ASA	5.9 ± 1.4 (384)	AAP	3.0 ± 1.1 (276)	0.07
AANA	9.6 ± 0.8 (1480)	ANA	7.6 ± 0.7 (1629)	0.03
AORN/T	7.7 ± 0.6 (2210)	ANA	7.6 ± 0.7 (1629)	0.47

Source: Cohen et al., 1974.

Table 4-7
Congenital Abnormality Rates (Skin Excluded) for Children of Wives of Male Respondents
All data adjusted for age and smoking habit, and all skin abnormalites were excluded. Rates are per 100 live births.

Organization	Rate	Organization	Rate	p
ASA	5.4 ± 0.4 (2988)	AAP	4.2 ± 0.5 (1714)	0.04
AANA	8.2 ± 0.9 (1168)	ANA	3.7 ± 2.5 (49)	0.13
AORN/T	6.4 ± 2.5 (203)	ANA	3.7 ± 2.5 (49)	0.22

Source: Cohen et al., 1974.

In reviewing the types of congenital abnormalities present among the offspring, a category of multifactorial inheritance was defined that included atrial septal defect, patent ductus, congenital hip, cleft palate or lip, clubfoot, pyloric stenosis, anencephaly, spina bifida, and hydrocephalus. When the abnormalty rates for these multifactorial abnormalities were compared in the children of operating room-exposed and operating room-unexposed physician groups, it was found that the differences in these special multifactorial categories were greater than those in the general anomaly group (Table 4-8). These differences give support to the suggestion that the increased risk of congenital abnormalities observed among children of operating room personnel may be influenced by environmental factors, as well as by genetic differences.

Table 4-8
Congenital Abnormality Rates Using Selected Multifactorial Categories
Categories include atrial septal defect, patent ductus, congenital hip, clubfoot, cleft palate or lip, pyloric stenosis, anencephaly, spina bifida, and hydrocephalus. Rates are per 100 live births.

	ASA	AAP	p
Female respondents	1.24 ± 0.47 (384)	0.21 ± 0.21 (276)	0.06
Wives of male respondents	1.56 ± 0.21 (2998)	0.90 ± 0.24 (1714)	0.03

Source: Cohen et al., 1974

Of additional concern, the study also revealed a significant increase in the occurrence of cancer[3] in operating room-exposed female

---

[3]These data were obtained from women respondents who reported that they presently were suffering from cancer or had been cured of their disease. Since no respondents were available, cancer deaths were not included.

respondents compared to control. The increase in cancer rates ranged from 1.3-fold to slightly less than 2-fold, with the highest rates found in both physician anesthetists and nurse anesthetists. A lesser increase in cancer incidence was noted among members of the operating room nurses/technicians group (Table 4-9).

Table 4-9
Cancer Incidence for Female Respondents
Data are age standardized, and skin cancers have been excluded.
Rates are per 100 respondents.

Organization	Rate	Organization	Rate	p
ASA	3.0 ± 0.6 (1008)	AAP	1.6 ± 0.5 (566)	0.05
AANA	2.6 ± 0.2 (6407)	ANA	1.8 ± 0.2 (5400)	<0.01
AORN/T	2.3 ± 0.2 (11843)	ANA	1.8 ± 0.2 (5400)	0.07

Source: Cohen et al., 1974.

Although precise data are not available, these findings suggest the possibility of a dose-response relationship with respect to the incidence of cancer in females and levels of anesthetic exposure for women who work in the operating room. Thus, female physician anesthetists evidence the largest increase in cancer rate. This finding may be associated with their long periods of exposure to the highest concentrations of waste anesthetic gases.

Analysis by type and location of cancer indicated no significant differences, with the exception of the incidences of leukemia and lymphoma which were increased approximately threefold in female respondents exposed to the operating room ($p = 0.05$). There was no increase in the incidence of cancer noted among exposed male respondents.

Hepatic disease was reported more frequently in all exposed respondent groups, both male and female, compared to control. After excluding serum hepatitis (operating room personnel have a high exposure to blood and blood products), the range of increase was 1.3- to 2.2-fold. Exposed male physician anesthetists showed a 58% increase in liver disease, and female anesthetists a 69% increase over their respective pediatric-physician control. These relative increases in liver disease, although statistically significant, are probably under-estimated since exposed female nurse anesthetists evidenced a 124% increase in liver disease (3.8% compared to only 1.7% for general duty nurses). The rate of liver disease in the control group of general duty nurses was significantly lower than that reported for the control group of female pediatricians (2.9%). This high incidence of liver disease in the pediatric group tended to skew the data and may reflect the unusually high exposure of pediatricians to viral infections (Table 4-10).

Table 4-10
Hepatic Disease Rates for Female Respondents
Cases of serum hepatitis have been excluded. Rates are per 100 respondents.

Organization	Rate	Organization	Rate	p
ASA	4.9 ± 0.7 (924)	AAP	2.9 ± 0.8 (512)	0.04
AANA	3.8 ± 0.3 (5178)	ANA	1.7 ± 0.2 (4512)	< 0.01
AORN/T	2.1 ± 0.2 (9741)	ANA	1.7 ± 0.2 (4512)	0.08

Source: Cohen et al., 1974.

Renal disease—pyelonephritis and cystitis excluded—was reported to be increased 1.2- to 1.4-fold in operating room-exposed female respondents compared to their control group. These differences, however, proved statistically significant only for the nurse anesthetists and operating room nurses/technicians (Table 4-11). There was no increase in the risk of renal disease among male physician anesthetists.

Despite these positive findings, which indicated an increased incidence of health hazards in operating room-exposed personnel, the authors were careful to point out that the study does not by itself establish a cause-and-effect relationship between reported increased disease rates and specific exposure to the waste anesthetic gases. Although anesthetic exposure provides a reasonable explanation for the observed increase in health problems, other unknown hazards may also be present in these locations. It is possible that certain of

Table 4-11
Renal Disease Rates for Female Respondents
Cases of pyelonephritis and cystitis have been excluded. Rates are
per 100 respondents.

Organization	Rate	Organization	Rate	p
ASA	2.4 ± 0.5 (908)	AAP	1.9 ± 0.7 (506)	0.28
AANA	3.1 ± 0.2 (5216)	ANA	2.3 ± 0.2 (4550)	0.01
AORN/T	2.9 ± 0.2 (9960)	ANA	2.3 ± 0.2 (4550)	0.05

Source: Cohen et al., 1974.

these undetermined factors may in turn have been responsible for the observed results.

An independent survey by Corbett et al. (1974) analyzed birth defects among offspring of Michigan female nurse anesthetists. In a survey of 621 nurse anesthetists, these authors found that 16.4% of mothers who worked during pregnancy produced children with birth defects, whereas only a 5.7% incidence of birth defects was observed among children of anesthetist mothers who did not work during their pregnancy (Table 4-12). Excluding skin anomalies, the incidences of major birth defects in the two groups were found to be 8.8% and 3.8%, respectively. These data are statistically significant.

Two smaller-scale epidemiologic studies were also conducted the same year. These were reported by Garstka, Wagner, and Hamacher (1974) in Germany and by Uhlirova and Pokorny (1974) in Czechoslovakia. In the German study, replies received from 257 anesthesiologists indicated significant increases in spontaneous abortion rates among female anesthesiologists (17.9%) compared to the same group before exposure of either parent to the operating room (10.6%). Congenital abnormalities in their children were significantly increased between the two groups before and after employment in the operating room (8.0% vs 1.5%). The rate of premature births among exposed female anesthetists was unusually high (19.7%), and pregnancy complications significantly increased among exposed female anesthesiologists (8.0%) compared to control (1.5%). Unfortunately, as in the earlier study by Askrog and Harvald (1970), no allowance was made for the increasing age of the mothers during the

Table 4-12
Incidence of Birth Defects Among Children of Practicing and Nonpracticing Michigan Nurse Anesthetists Compared to the Anomalies in Children of Nonanesthetists

	No. Respondents	No. Birth Anomalies	Percent Anomalies
Nurse anesthetists			
Working	434	81	16.4*
Nonworking	261	15	5.7
Nonanesthetists	5530	465	8.4

Source: Corbett et al., *Anesthesiology* 41:341–344, 1974. Reprinted by permission of the publisher, J.B. Lippincott, and of the author.
*$p < 0.01$ working nurse anesthetists versus nonworking nurse anesthetists, and working nurse anesthetists versus nonanesthetists.

period of study. The report from Czechoslovakia was based on a survey of 857 physicians, nurses, and technicians working in operating and recovery rooms. Although no control groups were provided, the authors reported an increased number of health problems with increasing years of service. Headache, fatigue, and allergic disease were noted, and the spontaneous abortion rate among women with more than five years of service in the anesthesia department was 8.1% compared to 4.8% among individuals with less than five years of service.

A preliminary survey of health hazards among dentists has also been reported by the ASA Ad Hoc Committee (Cohen et al., 1975). A mail survey of 4797 general dental practitioners and 2642 oral surgeons indicated that 20.2% of the general practitioners and 74.8% of the oral surgeons had anesthetic exposures in the dental operatory exceeding three hours per week. When a comparison was made of the health histories of individuals exposed and unexposed to inhalation anesthetics, there were significant increases in health problems among those dentists who used anesthetics in their practice. There was a 78% increase of spontaneous abortion in their spouses and a 156% increase in liver disease among the anesthetic-exposed dentists compared to control (serum hepatitis excluded) (Table 4-13). Small increases in congenital abnormality rates were recorded among exposed male dentists' children, and a small increase in cancer rate was also found in the exposed dentists. These differences, however, did not achieve statistical significance.

Table 4-13
Standardized Spontaneous Abortion Rates per 100 Pregnancies, Congenital Abnormality Rates per 100 Live-Born Babies, and Disease Rates per 100 Respondents in Anesthetic-Exposed versus Anesthetic-Unexposed Dentists

	Anesthetic-Exposed	Anesthetic-Unexposed	p
Spontaneous abortion (spouses)	16.0 ± 1.8 (887)	9.0 ± 1.0 (1541)	< 0.01
Liver disease	5.9 ± 0.4 (1528)	2.3 ± 0.4 (1249)	< 0.01
Congenital abnormalities	4.7 ± 1.1 (765)	4.1 ± 0.4 (1393)	0.26
Cancer	0.69 ± 0.26 (1631)	0.51 ± 0.18 (1326)	0.26

Source: Cohen et al., *J Am Dent Assoc.* 90:1291–1296, 1975. Copyright by the American Dental Association. Reprinted by permission.

Despite the limited scope of this preliminary dental survey, it is of particular interest because both general dentists and oral surgeons provide similar care to their patients in the dental operatory whether local or inhalation anesthetics are used. Yet, assignment of these individuals into one group exposed to anesthetic gases and a second group not so exposed reveals significant differences in disease rates. In comparing these data with results obtained for operating room physicians, the authors suggested that increases in certain health hazards among dentists may relate to the higher levels of exposure to waste anesthetic gases present in the dental operatory. These levels are customarily several times greater than those found in hospital operating rooms.

A study of anesthetic practice and pregnancy was carried out by Knill-Jones, Newman, and Spence (1975) among 7949 male physicians in the United Kingdom. This study represented a followup of an earlier survey of female physicians (Knill-Jones et al., 1972). Although paternal anesthetist exposure to the operating room exerted no apparent influence on the frequency of spontaneous abortion compared to control, maternal exposure was associated with a higher abortion rate than when neither parent was exposed (Table 4-14). The differences were further increased when pregnancies were carefully matched for maternal age, smoking habit, and child's birth order. Under these conditions, the frequency of spontaneous abortions was 14.9% among operating room-exposed women compared to 5.5% in the nonexposed group.

Table 4-14
Spontaneous Abortion Rates in Anesthetists or Spouses Exposed or Unexposed to the Operating Room During the First Trimester of Pregnancy

	No. Pregnancies	No. Spontaneous Miscarriages	Miscarriages/ Pregnancies (%)
Paternal exposure	5891	657	11.1
Maternal exposure	166	30	18.0*
No paternal or maternal exposure	7296	795	10.9

Source: Knill-Jones, Newman, and Spence, *Lancet* 2:807–809, 1975.
*p < 0.01.

Examination of congenital abnormality rates in male anesthetists' children indicated a significant increase compared to those in children born to nonoperating room-exposed male physicians. A somewhat higher incidence of congenital abnormalities was found in children of the operating room-exposed female anesthetist compared to control. However, most of these differences were accounted for by an increase in minor anomalies (Table 4-15). No significant differences were found in the types of congenital abnormalities among offspring whether there was no parental exposure, or whether one or both parents had been exposed to the operating room during the first trimester. There were also no differences in stillbirth rates.

In contrast to the results of the earlier Knill-Jones et al. report (1972) of a twofold increase in infertility among operating room-exposed female physicians, no significant differences were noted, in the present study, with regard to female fertility.

A small-scale survey by Mirakhur and Badve (1975), conducted in India, examined anesthetic practice and reproductive histories of 48 married female anesthetists, 50 nonanesthetist female physicians, wives of 136 anesthetists, and 47 male nonanesthetist physicians. Results of this survey indicated significant increases in spontaneous abortion rates among anesthetists (18.4%) compared to the other physicians (5.9%). There was a doubling in the incidence of congenital anomalies in children of operating room-exposed women

Table 4-15
Rates of Major and Minor Congenital Abnormalities in Children of Anesthetists or Spouses, Exposed and Unexposed to the Operating Room During the First Trimester of Pregnancy

	Total No. Children	Major Abnormality (%)	Minor Abnormality (%)	Total Abnormalities* (%)
Paternal exposure	5175	1.08 (56)	3.09† (160)	4.5‡ (235)
Maternal exposure	438	1.59 (7)	3.19 (14)	5.5 (24)
No paternal or maternal exposure	6442	1.05 (68)	2.35 (152)	3.6 (233)

Source: Knill-Jones, Newman, and Spence, 1975.

*Included 35 anomalies unassigned to category.
†$p < 0.02$ exposed versus unexposed.
‡$p < 0.05$ exposed versus unexposed.

compared to control (3.9% vs 1.8%), although statistical validity was not achieved within the small study population. The incidence of congenital anomalies in children born to wives of exposed male anesthetists versus those born to wives of nonexposed male physicians appeared to be increased (2.1% vs 1.7%), although this difference also was not statistically significant. There was, however, a significant delay present in certain milestones of development in children of exposed anesthetists compared to control (7.0% vs 0.8%).

Pharoah, Nikki, and Ahlman (1977) reported results of a retrospective survey that investigated pregnancy outcomes among 5700 female doctors registered in England and Wales during the period 1950 to 1975. Although these women had not been selected on the basis of a history of exposure to anesthetic gases, their work location at the time of conception was recorded. The results demonstrated no significant difference in spontaneous miscarriage rates between anesthetists and other women physicians. On the other hand, an anesthetic appointment appeared to be associated with higher stillbirth rates, smaller babies, and increased numbers of congenital malformations of the cardiovascular system compared to nonanesthetist female physicians. The last two observations proved statistically significant, whereas the first did not. The authors suggest that failure to demonstrate an increased spontaneous abortion rate among the anesthetists in their study may reflect the varying lengths of operating room exposure, which were not specifically investigated.

Spence, Cohen, and Brown (1977) undertook a comparative analysis of the health data obtained from three large studies of operating room-based physicians previously conducted in the United States (Cohen et al., 1974) and the United Kingdom. (Knill-Jones et al., 1972, 1975). Despite differences in population base, survey methods, and statistical analyses, there was remarkable agreement noted in the conclusions drawn from these independent studies. The combined group of 1333 pregnant U.S. and U.K. operating room-exposed female anesthetists showed a miscarriage rate significantly different from that of the 1909 unexposed control physicians (16.7% vs 13.3%) (Table 4-16). Similarly, the congenital abnormality rate in children born to the group of U.S. and U.K. operating room-exposed female anesthetists was significantly greater than that of the children born to control physicians (5.5% vs 4.0%). Analysis of the combined data of male physicians showed no difference in the spontaneous miscarriage rate in 5525 pregnancies among wives of exposed male anesthetists compared to 4754 pregnancies among wives of unexposed control physicians. On the other hand, the incidence of congenital abnormalities in children born to the operating room-exposed male anesthetists was significantly greater than that for the children born to unexposed male physicians (5.0% vs 3.7%).

Table 4-16
Adjusted and Combined Miscarriage and Congenital Abnormality Rates in Operating Room-Exposed Anesthetists in the United States and United Kingdom Compared to Unexposed Control Physicians

	No. Pregnancies	Miscarriages/Pregnancies (%)	No. Live-Born Children	Congenital Abnormalities/ Live-Born Children (%)
Exposed female anesthetists				
United States	596	15.7 ± 1.5	494	5.5 ± 1.0
United Kingdom	737	17.5 ± 1.4	599	5.5 ± 0.7
Combined	1333	16.7 ± 1.0*	1093	5.5 ± .07†
Unexposed female anesthetists				
United States	355	9.6 ± 1.6	313	2.8 ± 1.9
United Kingdom	2150	14.0 ± 0.8	1817	4.2 ± 0.4
Combined	2505	13.3 ± 0.7	2130	4.0 ± 0.4

Exposed male anesthetists				
United States	4143	12.1 ± 0.5	3597	5.3 ± 0.4
United Kingdom	1382	13.9 ± 0.9	1180	4.2 ± 0.7
Combined	5525	12.6 ± 0.5	4777	5.0 ± 0.3*
Unexposed male anesthetists				
United States	2261	12.0 ± 0.7	1970	3.9 ± 0.4
United Kingdom	3493	11.5 ± 0.6	2174	3.6 ± 0.4
Combined	4754	11.7 ± 0.5	4144	3.7 ± 0.3

Source: Spence, Cohen, and Brown, *JAMA*. 238:959, 1977. Copyright 1977, American Medical Association.

*p < 0.01 exposed versus unexposed.
†p < 0.04 exposed versus unexposed.

The authors also provided a comparative analysis of occupational diseases among male respondents in the two countries (Table 4-17). The age-adjusted cancer rates in the United States and the United Kingdom were similar for male operating room-exposed and operating room-unexposed physicians. Liver disease rates, however, were significantly greater in operating room-exposed male anesthetists in both countries than among their respective control physician groups.

Table 4-17
Adjusted Disease Rates for Exposed Male Anesthetists and Unexposed Control Physicians in the United States and the United Kingdom
Rates are per 100 respondents.

	United Kingdom		United States	
	A	N	A	P
No. respondents	1407	3502	5828	2337
Arrhythmias	0.07§	0.30	0.75	0.70
Cancer*	0.70§	0.79	0.70	0.70
Disc disease	1.44§	0.53	1.27	1.47
Gallbladder	1.34§	0.48	0.93	0.99
Hypertension	1.80§	0.80	2.31	2.47
Kidney disease†	1.70	2.10	4.20	4.60
Liver disease	3.09‡	1.79	4.90§	2.60
Migraine	0.15	0.00	0.23‡	0.06
Myocardial infarction	1.72	1.78	1.75	1.61
Peptic ulcer	2.30§	1.20	1.95	1.67
Ulcerative colitis	0.32	0.24	0.24‡	0.08
Renal lithiasis	1.27	1.14	3.07	3.27

A = Anesthetists   N = Nonanesthetists   P = Pediatricians

Source: Spence, Cohen, and Brown,*JAMA*. 238:955–959, 1977. Copyright 1977, American Medical Association.

*Excluding skin cancer.
†Excluding pyelonephritis.
‡$p < 0.01$ exposed versus unexposed.
§$p < 0.05$ exposed versus unexposed.

Of interest, although significant increases in the incidence of peptic ulcer, gallbladder disease, arterial hypertension, cardiac arrhythmia, and lumbar disc disease were present in operating room-exposed anesthetists in the United Kingdom compared to control, these differences were not present in the United States physician population. No differences were noted between anesthetists and other physicians in both countries with respect to the incidence of renal disease. There was, however, an approximate threefold increase in the overall reporting of renal disease in the United States compared to the physician groups in the United Kingdom. This difference was due almost entirely to an increased incidence of renal lithiasis among United States male physicians.

A limited survey conducted by Tomlin (1978) investigated the incidence in Birmingham of congenital abnormalities present in 135 children born to operating room-exposed anesthetists. A distinct pattern of serious congenital abnormalities was noted in 5 children in this group who evidenced defects confined to the musculoskeletal or nervous systems. Curiously, all of these abnormal children were female. The author suggested that the presence of 5 seriously affected children in only 75 families was likely the result of statistical clustering, although no control data were provided.

In a recent Finnish study, Rosenberg and Vanttinen (1978) examined reproductive hazards in anesthetists as compared to pediatricians. They reported a spontaneous miscarriage rate in 266 pregnancies among female pediatricians and wives of male pediatricians not working in the operating room which averaged 13.2%. This figure compared to the slightly higher 10.2% rate found in 252 pregnancies among female anesthetists and wives of working male anesthetists. Smoking mothers in both the pediatric and anesthetist groups had higher miscarriage rates. Congenital birth malformations occurred equally in children of both anesthetist and pediatric groups, although there was a particularly high incidence of musculoskeletal deformity among anesthetists' children. Despite the small data base, these authors concluded that their findings do not indicate that anesthetic gas pollution in the operating room is harmful to personnel.

A multiple logistic regression analysis of 12,914 pregnancies and 10,532 live births based on data from the ASA National Study (Cohen et al., 1974) was recently utilized by Himmelberger, Brown, and Cohen (1978) to assess the relationships between maternal cigarette smoking, spontaneous abortion, and congenital abnormalities. The data indicated that the risk of both spontaneous abortion and of congenital abnormality was significantly increased in smoking mothers. Women who smoked heavily before and during the first trimester of pregnancy had an estimated 1.2- to 1.7-fold increase in the rate of spontaneous abortion. The congenital abnormality rate among children born to these smoking mothers was 1.8 to 2.3 times greater than that among children of nonsmoking mothers, depending upon factors of age, previous pregnancy history, and exposure to the operating room. Operating room exposure proved an important additive contribution to the factor of smoking in the increase of both spontaneous abortion and congenital abnormalities. Thus, women at highest risk were those who smoked and were also exposed to the operating room prior to pregnancy and during the first trimester. However, the relative increase in miscarriage risk due to smoking was highest in women unexposed to the operating room.

Recently, a large national survey was initiated to examine the health of dental professionals in the United States. Although this study is still in progress, preliminary results indicate the presence of significant health problems among dentists exposed to anesthetics (Cohen et al., in preparation). The dental population offers unique advantages to study health effects associated with chronic exposure to trace anesthetic gases because: (1) the study population is large, in excess of 100,000 male dentists and 150,000 female chairside assistants; (2) the population is readily divided into an anesthetic-exposed group and a nonanesthetic-exposed control group, with the former using inhalation anesthetics in their practice and the latter working in similar dental operatories using only intravenous sedatives and local anesthetics; (3) the level of exposure to high concentrations of the waste anesthetics in the dental operatories is at least two to three times greater than that found in hospital operating rooms; (4) a significant number of dentists employing inhalation anesthetics limit their practice to the use of nitrous oxide, permitting separate analysis of this anesthetic.

The present study utilized two mail questionnaires and a telephone followup to survey a large random sample of the dentists and their chairside assistants. At the present writing, the questionnaire return rate is 73.6% for the dentists and approximately 73.3% for chairside assistants. Preliminary analysis of the data suggests that male members of the American Dental Association who use anesthetic gases in their dental operatory a minimum of nine hours per week show an increased incidence of liver disease, kidney disease, and general neurologic disease compared to the nonanesthetic-exposed control group (Table 4-18). The incidence of cancer appears identical for the exposure groups. The rate of spontaneous abortion in wives of the heavily anesthetic-exposed dentists is significantly increased, although the number of congenital abnormalities in their children is similar to that of control (Table 4-19).

Table 4-18
Incidence of Liver Disease, Kidney Disease, Neurologic Disease, and Cancer in Male Dentists
Exposure to the dental operatory was a minimum of nine hours per week. Rates are per 100 respondents and are adjusted for age and for smoking.

	Anesthetic Users	Nonanesthetic Users	p
Liver Disease	3.2 ± 0.29 (4517)	1.9 ± 0.16 (8386)	<0.01
Kidney disease	2.9 ± 0.26 (4516)	2.4 ± 0.18 (8387)	0.05
Neurologic disease	3.6 ± 0.29 (4517)	1.9 ± 0.15 (8387)	<0.01
Cancer	0.8 ± 0.15 (4515)	0.7 ± 0.09 (8383)	0.30

Source: Cohen et al., in preparation.

Table 4-19
Spontaneous Abortion and Congenital Abnormality Rates in Wives and Children of Male Dentists
Rates are per 100 live births and are adjusted for age and for smoking. Exposure to the dental operatory was a minimum of nine hours per week during year preceding event. Skin abnormalities have been excluded.

	Anesthetic Users Male Dentists	Nonanesthetic Users Male Dentists	p
Spontaneous abortion	10.2 ± 0.96 (1328)	6.7 ± 0.34 (5709)	<0.01
Congenital abnormalities	4.5 ± 0.63 (1177)	4.6 ± 0.29 (5277)	0.50

Source: Cohen et al., in preparation.

The female membership of the American Dental Association is relatively small (less than 2%), and thus data regarding health problems in female dental personnel have been limited to the chairside assistants. Preliminary data in Table 4-20 show significant health problems in chairside assistants associated with exposure to the anesthetic gases. The incidence of spontaneous abortion and possible congenital abnormalities appears greater in children of women exposed for nine or more hours per week to inhalation anesthetics in the year preceding the event (Table 4-20). As with male dentists, anesthetic exposure in the dental operatory also influences the incidence of liver disease. kidney disease, and general neurologic disease in these women (Table 4-21). Significant increases in the incidence of these health conditions are noted in female chairside assistants who work where inhalation anesthetics are employed. The preliminary data also suggest a marginally significant increase in the incidence of cancer among anesthetic-exposed women. This incidence is less than that previously reported in female operating room personnel (Cohen et al., 1974). Since the mean age of female dentists and chairside assistants was 29.7 years compared to 39.6 years for female operating room personnel, the normal incidence of cancer at these two age levels could account for the observed difference (Doll, 1976).

Data regarding use of various anesthetic agents in the dental operatory are provided in Table 4-22. Nitrous oxide is used as the exclusive anesthetic agent in 81.3% of cases, and in combination with potent agents in 18.7% of administrations. Of interest, an increased incidence of health problems is observed in both anesthetic groups. Table 4-23 provides data regarding spontaneous miscarriage in anesthetic-exposed versus nonanesthetic-exposed female chairside assistants. This information suggests that this health problem may be associated with the use of nitrous oxide alone. The possibility that the potent agents by themselves may produce an additive or synergistic response remains to be defined.

The effect of length of exposure in the operating room on the incidence of associated health problems is difficult to define. In the case of cancer, increased incidence may become apparent only after an exposure period of 20 years or more. Recently published data consider the effect of length of operating room exposure upon the incidence of obstetrical problems (Cohen, in press). Exposure of a pregnant woman during the first trimester of her pregnancy results in only a slight, not statistically significant, increase in spontaneous abortion and in congenital abnormality rates. However, if one adds to this first-trimester operating room exposure the factor of a previous long-term exposure of at least one year preceding pregnancy, the risk of spontaneous abortion and congenital abnormalities increases significantly.

Table 4-20
Spontaneous Abortion Rates and Congenital Abnormality Rates in Children of Female Chairside Assistants
Rates are per 100 live births and are adjusted for age and for smoking. Exposure to the dental operatory was a minimum of nine hours per week during year preceding the event. Skin abnormalities have been excluded.

	Anesthetic Users	Nonanesthetic Users	p
Spontaneous abortion	19.1 ± 20 (400)	8.1 ± 0.48 (3184)	<0.01
Congenital abnormalities	4.9 ± 1.2 (316)	3.6 ± 0.34 (2882)	0.20

Source: Cohen et al., in preparation.

Table 4-21
Incidence of Liver Disease, Kidney Disease, Nonspecific Neurologic Disease, and Cancer in Female Chairside Assistants
Exposure to the dental operatory was a minimum of nine hours per week. Rates are per 100 respondents and are adjusted for age and for smoking.

	Anesthetic Users	Nonanesthetic Users	p
Liver disease	1.6 ± 0.22 (2738)	1.0 ± 0.12 (6924)	<,0.01
Kidney disease	4.1 ± 0.39 (2731)	2.4 ± 0.19 (6916)	<0.01
Neurologic disease	4.6 ± 0.43 (2740)	1.7 ± 0.15 (6926)	<0.01
Cancer	1.1 ± 0.18 (2733)	0.7 ± 0.10 (6920)	0.06

Source: Cohen et al., in preparation.

76

Table 4-22
Inhalation Anesthetic Agent Used in the Dental Operatory by Dentists and Chairside Assistants

N$_2$O alone	81.3%
*N$_2$O plus potent inhalation agent	18.7%

Source: Cohen et al., in preparation.

*Potent inhalation anesthetics include halothane, methoxyflurane, trichloroethylene, and enflurane.

Table 4-23
Incidence of Spontaneous Abortion in Chairside Assistants According to Anesthetic Usage
Rates are per 100 live births and are adjusted for age and for smoking.

	Spontaneous Miscarriage	p
Nonanesthetic users	8.5 ± 0.46 (3771)	
Nitrous oxide alone	16.1 ± 1.25 (893)	<0.01
Nitrous oxide plus potent inhalation agent	25.0 ± 4.33 (139)	<0.01

Source: Cohen et al., in preparation.

Of the two, long-term exposure appears to be the more significant factor (Figure 4-1).

Considering the long-term reproductive exposure risk, an important question is whether a woman should remain away from the operating room environment if she intends to become pregnant. Fortunately, the data suggest that both spontaneous miscarriage and congenital abnormality rates tend to return to normal after time away from the operating room (Figure 4-2). Return toward a normal spontaneous miscarriage rate, however, occurs more rapidly than does the return for congenital abnormalities. The latter finding would appear to dictate a woman's absence from the operating room for at least two years to reachieve baseline level.

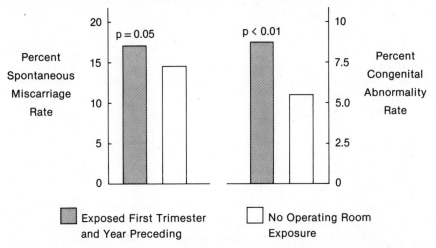

Figure 4-1 Spontaneous miscarriage and congenital abnormality rates among physicians and nurse anesthetists exposed to the operating room during the first trimester, plus one year preceding pregnancy. These data are compared to female anesthetists away from the operating room during a similar period. (From Cohen, in press)

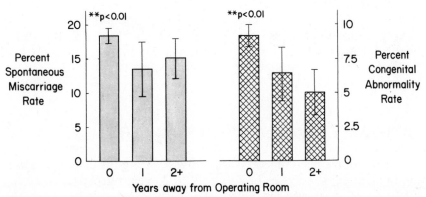

Figure 4-2 Return of spontaneous miscarriage and congenital abnormality rates to control level upon absence of the female anesthetist from the operating room. (From Cohen, in press)

Although there are important differences in design, conduct, and statistical analyses provided for the 20 various reported epidemiologic surveys, there appears to be majority agreement which indicates an increased hazard for spontaneous miscarriage among operating room-exposed females. The data on congenital abnormalities are less secure, but the two largest published studies provide significant information indicating an increased risk associated with maternal and/or paternal exposure. Data for an increased incidence of liver disease in operating room-exposed personnel also appear consistent. The data on cancer in females are limited to the United States study. Both the large United States and United Kingdom surveys found no increase in the incidence of cancer in males.

Finally, the results of an earlier small-scale dental survey have been confirmed in a more recent extensive national study which indicates significant increases in health hazards among dentists and chair-side personnel. This latter study offers strong evidence for causal association between these health findings and exposure to waste anesthetic gases in the workplace.

Although review of the preceding series of epidemiologic studies might lead the reader to conclude the established presence of a significant health hazard in the operating room or dental operatory and its likely association with waste anesthetic gases, one must bear in mind the limitations of the epidemiologic method. In a recent review of health hazards associated with anesthetic practice (Spence and Knill-Jones, 1978), the authors carefully pointed out that even in the large-scale operating room studies, reply rates have not been ideal, and it is virtually impossible to eliminate bias in reporting. In addition, although exposure of all individuals to the anesthetic agents was assumed to be equal, this represents an approximation since exposure was not actually measured. Another recent reviewer (Vessey, 1978), while accepting the evidence for increased spontaneous abortion among exposed females, found unconvincing evidence for other health hazards. Thus, despite the strength of the data presented, a level of caution in interpretation appears warranted.

MORTALITY AMONG ANESTHESIOLOGISTS

There have been several studies investigating the causes of death among United States anesthesiologists. A 20-year retrospective survey by Bruce et al. (1968) examined 441 deaths among members of the ASA during the period 1947 to 1966. Comparison of these death rates with Bureau of Vital Statistics data for males and with insurance company records indicates a lower incidence of lung cancer and coronary heart disease, a high suicide rate, and an increase in malignancies of the reticuloendothelial system among anesthesiologists. Although a strong trend was noted, especially for the last two findings, the data were not statistically significant, and the authors carefully pointed out the limitations of their retrospective information.

Bruce et al. (1974b), in a second study, reported results of a five-year prospective survey (1967 through 1971) covering 211 deaths among members of the ASA. Using methods of comparison similar to those employed in their earlier study (Bruce et al., 1968), the authors found that overall death rates were lower in anesthesiologists than in control groups with the exception of suicide (+ 197%). The previously suggested finding of an increased rate for malignancies of the lymphoid and reticuloendothelial tissues was not confirmed.

Doll and Peto (1977) examined mortality rates among doctors in different occupations with special emphasis on their smoking habits. Smoking habits for both anesthetists and part-time anesthetic users fell within the median range, as did their incidence of smoking-related disease. Although the findings were not statistically significant, anesthetists appeared to have lower rates of ischemic heart disease and myocardial degeneration, chronic bronchitis, emphysema, and pulmonary heart disease. Cancer of the pancreas was markedly greater among anesthetists, but this finding likely represented a chance finding in the small population tested.

Very recently, the American Cancer Society (Lew, 1979) has retrospectively examined mortality experience among active members of the ASA during the period 1954 through 1976. Data obtained from society files, plus examination of death certificates of 610 male anesthesiologists accredited prior to 1967, indicate that mortality among anesthesiologists from all causes was 84.1% of the expected death rate for all physicians. There was no evidence of an increased cancer death rate among male physicians. Cancer accounted for an average of 18.7% of all causes of deaths among anesthesiologists accredited prior to 1960, and for 20.6% of deaths in anesthesiologists of record in 1967. Rates for the control group were 19.5% and 20.0%, respectively. The suicide rate in male anesthesiologists approximated 6% of the total death rate, representing a fourfold increase over that expected. Study data for female anesthesiologists were too small to permit conclusions. However, 33 death certificates were available for examination, with 15 deaths attributed to cancer. The overall mortality rate among this small group of female anesthesiologists, however, was not increased compared to other female physicians.

EFFECT OF WASTE ANESTHETIC GASES ON
OPERATING ROOM PERFORMANCE

The hazards of surgery and anesthesia are significant, and the patient's immediate survival depends upon the alertness and performance of the professional team. Recent studies suggest that performance and alertness in the operating room may not necessarily always be maximal, and that under certain circumstances, accumulated concentrations of waste anesthetic gases may be sufficiently high so as to interfere with perceptual, cognitive, and motor skills of the physicians and nurses who continually work in this environment.

Data have been presented for trichloroethylene, which is both an anesthetic and an industrial solvent. The TLV (threshold-limiting value) for industrial application has been set at 100 ppm. Salvini, Binaschi, and Riva (1971) reported that exposure of six male volunteers to trichloroethylene concentrations of 110 ppm for two four-hour periods resulted in significant decreases in performance measured by both perceptual and dexterity tests. The authors concluded that the defined TLV concentrations are too high to prevent interference with psychological efficiency in the workplace. Recent studies (Corbett et al., 1973a) indicate that the defined critical concentrations of trichloroethylene are exceeded within 4 feet of the expiratory valve of the anesthesia machine during clinical administrations of this anesthetic.

Bruce, Bach, and Arbit (1974a) examined the effects of trace concentrations of both nitrous oxide and halothane on psychological performance. Forty male students were exposed on each of two occasions to four-hour inhalations of either air alone or air combined with 500 ppm nitrous oxide with or without 15 ppm halothane. These trace anesthetic concentrations have been reported as present in unscavenged operating rooms. During experimental exposure, the subject was seated in a reclining chair over which an oxygen tent was suspended for administration of air or anesthetic. Immediately after exposure, the subject was given a battery of tests which measured perceptual, cognitive, and motor skills. Comparison of responses from subjects breathing air and those exposed to halothane and nitrous oxide indicate significant decrements in performance among those receiving the anesthetic (Table 4-24). Of interest, 6 of 20 subjects fell asleep at some time during the four-hour period, and in each instance, sleep occurred in the anesthetic exposure situation.

Subsequently, Bruce and Bach (1975) exposed an additional 30 male subjects under similar circumstances to 500 ppm nitrous oxide and 15 ppm enflurane in air. Performance on a divided-attention

Table 4-24
Significance Values for Test Performance Differences in Volunteer Subjects after Exposure to 15 ppm Halothane and 500 ppm N₂O in Air Compared to Control Subjects Breathing Room Air.

Task	p
Audiovisual task	< 0.01
Tachistoscopic task	± 0.025
Memory passages	< 0.05
Digit span	< 0.05

Source: Bruce, Bach, and Arbit, *Anesthesiology* 40:453–458, 1974a. Reprinted by permission of the publisher, J.B. Lippincott, and of the author.

audiovisual task and a digit-span memory task was significantly decreased in the anesthetized subjects compared to those subjects breathing air. Performance on the tachistoscopic task and tests from the Wechsler memory and intelligence scale, however, was not affected. An additional group of subjects exposed to 500 ppm nitrous oxide in air alone scored significantly lower only on the digit-span test. The authors concluded that the trace concentrations of anesthetics present in unscavenged operating rooms may interfere with optimum performance.

Further studies by Bruce and Bach (1976) evaluated the effect of concentrations of nitrous oxide and halothane as low as 50 ppm and 1 ppm, respectively. These concentrations produced measurable decrements in performance on psychological tests in healthy, male volunteers. Nitrous oxide alone also produced a diminished response. Functions most sensitive to these low concentrations of anesthetics were visual perception, immediate memory, and a combination of perception, cognition, and motor responses required in a task of divided attention to simultaneous visual and auditory stimuli. No decrements in performance were present in subjects exposed to concentrations of nitrous oxide 25 ppm and halothane 0.5 ppm.

Gamberale and Svensson (1974) examined the effect of anesthetic gases on psychomotor and perceptual function in two groups of Swedish nurses. Twenty anesthetic nurses and 20 nurses with duties in the intensive care unit were tested with respect to reaction times and perceptual speed at the start and end of a workday. The anesthetic nurses were exposed daily to anesthetic gases usually present in the air during their workday in several hospitals. Halothane concentrations varied between 0.5 and 10 ppm and nitrous oxide concentrations from 30 to 3000 ppm. No measurable impairment in reaction time and in perceptual speed was noted among the anesthetic nurses compared to control, although results on one of the reaction time tests indicated that individual variability on the responses of the anesthetic nurses at the end of the workday was greater than that found in the comparison group (Figure 4-3).

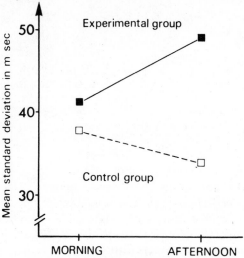

Figure 4-3 Mean values of individual standard deviations in simple reaction times for the experimental group (nurse anesthetists) and the control group (intensive care nurses) in the morning at the start of work and in the afternoon at the end of work. (From Gamgerale and Svensson, *Environ Health.* 11:108–119, 1974. Reprinted by permission of the *Scandinavian Journal of Work, Environment and Health.*)

Despite consistency of the preceding reports, these positive findings have not been confirmed by other investigators. Smith and Shirley (1977) examined the effects of nitrous oxide 500 ppm and halothane 15 ppm on psychomotor performance of 10 anesthetic technicians using audiovisual reaction time tests similar to those employed by Bruce and associates. No decrement in performance was noted following an exposure period of three to four hours.

Frankhuizen et al. (1978) studied 24 male subjects who breathed air or nitrous oxide 1600 ppm and halothane 16 ppm in air in two alternate two-hour sessions. Several psychomotor tests, including the highly sensitive audiovisual four-choice reaction time task were used. These measures failed to demonstrate any adverse effect from the trace anesthetics.

Most recently, Cook et al. (1978) examined 29 male students exposed to concentrations of halothane up to 200 ppm, concentrations of halothane 20 ppm plus nitrous oxide 500 ppm, and nitrous oxide alone 4000 ppm. None of these concentrations was found to influence tests of complex reaction time or immediate recall (digit span). Subanesthetic concentrations of nitrous oxide (20%) and halothane (0.2%), were, however, sufficient to impair mental function. Similar responses in altered decision-making behavior have been reported in volunteers following their inhalation of 0.25% enflurane (Bentin, Collins, and Adam, 1978).

Although certain nuances in experimental design may help to explain these conflicting data, the issue of performance potential in the presence of trace anesthetic gases presently remains unresolved despite its obvious clinical importance.

ENZYME INDUCTION AND ALTERATIONS OF THE IMMUNE RESPONSE IN ANESTHETISTS

The presence of measurable concentrations of volatile anesthetics in the blood and expired air of anesthetists has been confirmed from many sources (Hallen, Ehrner-Samuel, and Thomason, 1970; Whitcher, Cohen, and Trudell, 1971; Corbett and Ball, 1971; Pfaffli et al., 1972; Gostomyzk et al., 1975). It has been estimated that during a single year, the working anesthetist may absorb into his or her body the approximate equivalent of two full surgical anesthetics (25,000 to 30,000 ppm hours) (Gotell and Stahl, 1972). It is not surprising that these absorbed concentrations are associated with significant physiologic effects which, although not etiologically proven, may be causally associated with the increased incidence of spontaneous miscarriage, congenital abnormalities in children, liver disease, and female cancer observed among operating room-exposed personnel. In addition to these health hazards, other physiologic alterations in the operating room-exposed anesthetists have also been noted.

Induction of Drug-Metabolizing Enzymes

A large number of drugs and chemical compounds, possibly as many as 300, including the inhalation anesthetics, have been shown to stimulate activity of drug-metabolizing enzymes in liver microsomes. Several studies of anesthetists suggest that enzyme induction may also occur as a result of long-term operating room exposure. Cascorbi, Blake, and Helrick (1970) demonstrated that the urinary excretion of ^{14}C-labeled halothane metabolites following intravenous administration of a small dose of radioactive anesthetic was greater in four out of five anesthetists than in pharmacists, although statistical significance was not established. Neither group had been exposed to known agents capable of inducing drug-metabolizing enzymes, and the only obvious difference between groups was exposure of the anesthetists to an operating room atmosphere contaminated with anesthetics. After considering the wide variability in halothane metabolite excretion patterns noted in both anesthetists and controls, these workers conducted a follow-up examination in a previously tested anesthetist (Cascorbi, Blake, and Helrich, 1972). In this single individual, an additional year of occupational exposure to halothane was associated with a further increase in urinary metabolite excretion.

Evers and Racz (1974) published a preliminary study of blood enzymes, morphology, and serum proteins in anesthesia residents. Fifteen new residents were followed for periods of 12 to 48 months. During this time, there were increases in SGOT, SGPT, LDH, and alkaline phosphatase. Increases peaked between the ninth to eleventh months of training and then leveled off or returned to near normal values. Blood albumin levels frequently decreased, as did several of the globulin fractions.

Bardzik et al. (1975b) examined 22 anesthetists and anesthetic nurses who averaged 7.9 years of work experience. These researchers were unable to demonstrate significant increases in enzyme activity, serum bilirubin, or thymol turbidity in these anesthetists beyond control levels. In a few instances, however, slight abnormalities in alkaline phosphatase and in GGTP were noted.

An examination of drug-metabolizing ability among operating room personnel was also carried out by Wood, O'Malley, and Stevenson (1974) in 23 anesthetists and operating room technicians matched with a nonexposed control group. Determination of antipyrine clearance rates indicated the half life for the exposed group to average 11.1 ± 3.1 hours, and for the control group 12.7 ± 3 hours. These differences were statistically significant.

An interesting study by Ghoneim et al. (1975) investigated the plasma half-life of warfarin in a control group of five subjects and in seven anesthesia residents before beginning training and again four months after. The plasma half-lives in the control group remained essentially unchanged, whereas the half-life of the operating room-exposed residents was increased, as were the prothrombin responses (Table 4-25). None of the operating rooms to which the anesthesia residents were exposed had equipment for scavenging overflow anesthetics. Because warfarin is cleared from the plasma primarily by metabolism, changes in the plasma half-life of warfarin may be considered to reflect alterations in the rate of its metabolism by hepatic microsomal enzymes. The data suggest that exposure of an individual to the operating room environment is associated with changes in warfarin metabolism, with the most likely route through induction of drug-metabolizing enzymes.

Table 4-25
Plasma Half-Lives of Warfarin (Hours) and Prothrombin (Seconds)
Comparing Anesthesia Residents and a Control Group

	Plasma Half-Life		Prothrombin Time	
	Initial	4 Months Later	Initial	4 Months Later
Control subjects	38.8 ± 4.1	37.7 ± 2.6	1.670 ± 64	1.730 ± 96
Anesthesia residents	32.1 ± 3.6	$49.3 \pm 4.8^*$	1.337 ± 78	$1.552 \pm 22^*$

Source: Ghoneim et al., *Anesthesiology.* 43:333–336, 1975.
Reprinted by permission of the publisher, J.B. Lippincott, and of the author.

$^*p<0.05$ control versus operating room exposure.

Alterations in the Immune Response

Although there are data to indicate that general anesthesia in sufficient quantity may interfere with the immune response, Bruce (1972) was unable to demonstrate immunosuppression in anesthesiologists occupationally exposed to the operating room. PHA-stimulated lymphocytes obtained from six exposed anesthetists and six male student controls showed no evidence of lymphocyte stimulation. A more recent study (Harman et al., 1978) analyzed antipyrine kinetics in eight anesthetists alternatively exposed in the operating room or working exclusively in the intensive care unit (anesthetic-unexposed). Antipyrine half-life was reduced, and clearance increased during the period of exposure to waste anesthetic gases in the operating room.

Bardzik, Przezdziak, and Bardzik (1975a) investigated immunoglobulins in 18 anesthetists and anesthetic nurses, and whereas the levels of IgA and IgG were within normal range, the IgM level was raised in 15 out of 18 individuals. This statistically significant response was considered important in that immunoglobulin M is stimulated selectively by macromolecular antigens possessing multiple antigenic determinants in periodically repeated sequences.

Salo and Vapaavoun (1976), however, studied 10 healthy anesthetists who had been employed in the operating room for an average of 5.6 years and were concerned with the effect operating room exposure might have on their immune response. Using the rosette method, these authors found no differences in numbers of T- and B-lymphocytes among anesthetists and control.

It appears that the trace levels of anesthetics present in the operating room probably do not interfere significantly with the anesthetists' immune response.

Miscellaneous Adverse Physiologic Responses in Exposed Anesthetists

Several case reports attest to additional problems present in occupationally exposed anesthetists. These problems include exacerbation of subclinical myasthenia gravis in a nurse anesthetist exposed to methoxyflurane (Elder et al., 1971), delayed asthmatic attack following exposure to enflurane (Schwettmann and Casterline, 1976), atrial fibrillation in an anesthetist exposed to halothane (Lattey, 1970), laryngitis with headaches and lassitude following trace halothane exposure (Pitt, 1974), and excretion of trace concentrations of halothane in the breast milk of a lactating practicing anesthetist (Coté et al., 1976).

REFERENCES

Askrog, V., and Harvald, B. Teratogenic effects of inhalation anesthetics. *Nord Med.* 83:498–500, 1970.

Bardzik, J., Bardzik, I., Kryszewski, A., et al. Serum enzyme levels in anaesthetic personnel. *Anesth Resus Int Ther.* 4:291–295, 1975b.

Bardzik, J., Przezdziak, J., and Bardzik, I. Immunoglobulin in persons with long-term exposure to halothane. *Anesth Resus Int Ther.* 4:285–290, 1975a.

Bentin, S., Collins, G.I., and Adam, N. Decision-making behaviour during inhalation of subanaesthetic concentrations of enflurane. *Br J Anaesth.* 50:1173-1177, 1978.

Boyd, C.H. Ophthalmic hyper-sensitivity to anaesthetic vapour. *Anaesthesia.* 27:456-457, 1974.

Bruce, D.L. Eide, K.A., Linde, H.W., et al. Causes of death among anesthesiologists: A 20-year study. *Anesthesiology.* 29:565-569, 1968.

Bruce, D.L. Immunologically competent anesthesiologists. *Anesthesiology.* 37:76-78, 1972.

Bruce, D.L.,Bach, M.J., and Arbit, J. Trace anesthetic effects of perceptual, cognitive, and motor skills. *Anesthesiology.* 40:453-458, 1974a.

Bruce, D.L., Eide, K.A., Smith, N.J., et al. A prospective survey of anesthesiologist mortality, 1967-1971. *Anesthesiology.* 41:71-74, 1974b.

Bruce, D.L., and Bach, M.J. Psychological studies of human performance as affected by traces of enflurane and nitrous oxide. *Anesthesiology.* 42:194-196, 1975.

_____. Effects of trace anaesthetic gases on behavioural performance of volunteers. *Br J Anaesth.* 48:871-875, 1976.

Cascorbi, H.F., Blake, D.A., and Helrich, M. Differences in the biotransformation of halothane in man. *Anesthesiology.* 32:119-123, 1970.

_____. Halothane biotransformation in mice and man. Edited by B.R. Fink. In *Cellular Biology and Toxicity of Anesthetics.* Baltimore, Md.: Williams and Wilkins Company, 1972.

Cohen, E.N., Bellville, J.W., and Brown, B.W. Anesthesia, pregnancy, and miscarriage: A study of operating room nurses and anesthetists. *Anesthesiology.* 35:343-347, 1971.

Cohen, E.N., Brown, B.W., Bruce, D.L., et al. Occupational disease among operating room personnel: A national study. *Anesthesiology.* 41:321-340, 1974.

_____. A survey of anesthetic health hazards among dentists. *J Am Dent Assoc.* 90:1291-1296, 1975.

Cohen, E.N. Waste anesthetic gases and reproductive health in OR personnel. Edited by P. Infante. *Workshop on Methodology for Assessing Reproductive Hazards in the Workplace.* Washington, D.C.: 1979. (In press).

Cohen, E.N., Brown, B.W., Wu, M., et al. Survey of health hazards among dentists and dental assistants. (In preparation)

Cook, T.L., Smith, M., Starkweather, J.A., et al. Behavioral effects of trace and subanesthetic halothane and nitrous oxide in man. *Anesthesiology.* 49:419-424, 1978.

Corbett, T.H., and Ball, G.L. Chronic exposure to methoxy-flurane: A possible occupational hazard to anesthesiologists. *Anesthesiology.* 34:532–537, 1971.

Corbett, T.H., Hamilton, G.C., Yoon, M.K., et al. Occupational exposure of operating room personnel to trichloroethylene. *Can Anaesth Soc J.* 20:675–678, 1973a.

Corbett, T.H., Cornell, R.G., Lieding, K., et al. Incidence of cancer among Michigan nurse anesthetists. *Anesthesiology.* 38:260–263, 1973b.

Corbett, T.H., Cornell, R.G. Endres, J.L., et al. Birth defects among children of nurse-anesthetists. *Anesthesiology.* 41:341–344, 1974.

Corbett, T.H., Endres, J.L., et al. Birth defects among children of nurse-anesthetists. *Anesthesiology.* 41:341–344, 1974.

Coté, C.J., Kenepp, N.B., Reed, S.B., et al. Trace concentrations of halothane in human breast milk. *Br J Anaesth.* 48:541–543, 1976.

Doll, R. Cancer Incidence in Five Continents. Vol. III, Edited by Richard Doll. I.A.R.C. Scientific Publications, No. 15, Lyon, 1976.

Doll, R., and Peto, R. Mortality among doctors in different occupations. *Br Med J.* 2:1433–1436, 1977.

Elder, B.F., Beal, H., DeWald, W., et al. Exacerbation of subclinical myasthenia by occupational exposure to an anesthetic. *Anes Analog (Cleve)* 50:383–387, 1971.

Evers, W., and Racz, G.B. Occupational hazards in anesthesia: Survey of blood enzymes, morphology, and serum proteins in anesthesia residents. *Anesth Resus Int Ther.* 2:179–181, 1974.

Frankhuizen, J.L., Vlek, C.A.J., Burm, A.G.L., et al. Failure to replicate negative effects of trace anaesthetics on mental performance. *Br J Anaesth.* 50:229–234, 1978.

Gamberale, F., and Svensson, G. The effect of anesthetic gases on the psychomotor and perceptual functions of anesthetic nurses. *Scand J Work Environ Health.* 11:108–113, 1974.

Garstka, K., Wagner, K.L., and Hamacher, M. Complications of pregnancy in female anesthesiologists. *Geburtshilfe Frauenheilkd.* 35:826–833, 1974.

Ghoneim, M.M., Delle, M., Wilson, W. R., et al. Alteration of warfarin kinetics in man associated with exposure to an operating room environment. *Anesthesiology.* 43:333–336, 1975.

Gostomzyk, J.G., Frey, R., Gregori, M., et al. Die gafahrdung des operationssaal-personals durch narkosegase. *Diagnostik.* 8:403–407, 1975.

Gotell, P., and Stahl, R. Halothan-exposition hos narkosskoter-skor. *Lakartidningen.* 69:6179–6183, 1972.

Hallen, B., Ehrner-Samuel, H., and Thomason, M. Measurements of halothane in the atmosphere of operating theatre and in expired air and blood of the personnel during routine anaesthetic work. *Acta Anaesthesiol Scand.* 14:17–27, 1970.

Harman, A.W., Russell, W.J., Frewin, D.B., et al. Altered drug metabolism in anaesthetists exposed to volatile anaesthetic agents. *Anaesth Intensive Care.* 6:210-214, 1978.

Himmelberger, D.U., Brown, B.W., and Cohen, E.N. Cigarette smoking during pregnancy and the occurrence of spontaneous abortion and congenital abnormality. *Am J Epidemiol.* 108:470–479, 1978.

Knill-Jones, R.P., Moir, D.D., Rodrigues, L.V., et al. Anaesthetic practice and pregnancy; Controlled survey of women anaesthetists in the United Kingdom. *Lancet.* 2:1326–1328, 1972.

Knill-Jones, R.P., Newman, B.J., and Spence, A.A. Anaesthetic practice and pregnancy: Controlled survey of male anaesthetists in the United Kingdom. *Lancet.* 2:807–809, 1975.

Lattey, M. Halothane sensitization: A case report. *Can Anaesth Soc J.* 17:648–649, 1970.

Lew, E.A. Mortality experience among anesthesiologists, 1954–1976. *Anesthesiology.* (In press)

Mirakhur, R.K., and Badve, A.V. Pregnancy and anaesthetic practice in India. *Anaesthesia.* 30:18–22, 1975.

Pfaffli, P., Nikki, P., and Ahlman, K. Halothane and nitrous oxide in end-tidal air and venous blood of surgical personnel. *Ann Clin Res.* 4:273–277, 1972.

Pharoah, P.O.D., Alberman, E., and Doyle, R. Outcome of pregnancy among women in anaesthetic practice. *Lancet.* 1:34–36, 1977.

Pitt, E.M. Halothane as a possible cause of laryngitis in an anaesthetist. *Anaesthesia.* 29:579–580, 1974.

Rosenberg, P.H., and Kirves, A. Miscarriages among operating room staff. *Acta Anaesthesiol Scand.* 53(suppl):37–42, 1973.

Rosenberg, P.H., and Vanttinen, H. Occupational hazards to reproduction and health in anaesthetists and paediatricians. *Acta Anaesthesiol Scand.* 22:202–207, 1978.

Salo, M., and Vapaavoun, M. Peripheral blood T- and B-lymphocytes in operating theatre personnel. *Br J Anaesth.* 48:877–886, 1976.

Salvini, M., Binaschi, S., and Riva, M. Evaluation of the psychophysiological functions in humans exposed to trichloroethylene. *Br J Ind Med.* 28:293–295, 1971.

Schwettmann, R.S., and Casterline, C.L. Delayed asthmatic response following occupational exposure to enflurane.

Anesthesiology. 44:166–169, 1976.

Smith, G., and Shirley, A.W. Failure to demonstrate effect of trace concentrations of nitrous oxide and halothane on psychomotor performance. *Br J Anaesth.* 49:65–70, 1977.

Spence, A.A., Cohen, E.N., and Brown, B.W. Occupational hazards for operating room-based physicians. Analysis of data from the United States and United Kingdom. *JAMA.* 238:955–959, 1977.

Spence, A.A., and Knill-Jones, R.P. Is there a health hazard in anaesthetic practice? *Br J Anaesth.* 50:713–719, 1978.

Tomlin, P.J. Teratogenic effects of waste anesthetic gases. *Br Med J.* 1:108, 1978.

Uhlirova, A., and Pokorny, J. Results of questionnaire survey of health of anesthesiologists. *Rozhl Chir.* 53:761–770, 1974.

Vaisman, A.I. Working conditions in surgery and their effect on health of anesthesiologists. *Eksp Khir Anestheziol.* 3:44–49, 1967.

Vessey, M.P. Epidemiological studies of the occupational hazards of anaesthesia: A review. *Anaesthesia.* 33:430–438, 1978.

Whitcher, C.E., Cohen, E.N., and Trudell, J.R. Chronic exposure to anesthetic gases in the operating room. *Anesthesiology.* 35:348–353, 1971.

Wood, M., O'Malley, K., and Stevenson, I.H. Drug metabolizing ability in operating theatre personnel. *Br J Anaesth.* 46:726–728, 1974.

5 Mechanisms of Toxicity

It has been well documented that acute and/or long-term toxicity may follow the clinical administration of an anesthetic. Almost ironically, we now realize that it is not the patient alone who is at risk from this anesthetic administration. Measurements in the operating room indicate that during conduct of a clinical anesthetic, concentrations of anesthetic gases continuously escape into the room air. Thus, operating room personnel (i.e., nurses, surgeons, and anesthetists) are exposed to and constantly rebreathe trace concentrations of anesthetics. Although the absorbed concentrations of these anesthetics are low, they are nonetheless sufficient to produce significant physiologic alterations.

It has been suggested (Fink and Cullen 1976) that chronic exposure to trace anesthetic concentrations may offer lesser hazard than briefer exposure at an anesthetizing concentration, even if equivalent amounts of anesthetic agent (MAC hours) are administered. Although indefinite exposure to subnarcotic concentrations can never produce the anesthetic state, chronic exposure to subanesthetic concentrations results in sustained blood anesthetic levels, induction of drug-metabolizing enzymes, and increased biodegradation of the anesthetic (Berman and Bochantin, 1970; Rietbrock, Lazarus, and Otterbein, 1972). Anesthetic metabolism with resultant formation of reactive intermediary species is known to be associated with a significant increase in toxicity (Scholler, 1970; Stevens et al., 1975; Mazze, Hitt, and Cousins, 1974; Sipes and Brown, 1976; etc.).

As indicated earlier, epidemiologic studies of female operating room nurses and anesthetists indicate an increased spontaneous miscarriage rate among women occupationally exposed to the operating room. Several additional studies suggest even more serious problems, including congenital abnormalities in offspring and an increase in cancer in females. Rates of hepatic disease also appear to be significantly higher in both male and female operating room-exposed personnel.

The precise etiologic mechanism(s) involved in these untoward health responses have not been defined. There is, however, evidence to support several hypotheses. These hypotheses include the possibilities of direct depressant action of inhalation anesthetics on cell growth, cell injury resulting from formation and covalent binding of reactive anesthetic metabolites, the presence of specialized hazards in the operating room including various chemicals, x-ray, oncotic viruses, and the possibility of stress-induced abnormality and disease.

EFFECTS OF ANESTHETICS ON CELL GROWTH

Anesthetics have long been known to produce depression of cell growth. Bernard (1878) reported a century ago that placement of an ether-soaked sponge within a bell jar retards the growth of seedlings, implying an arrest of cell division (Figure 5-1). Subsequent studies by other workers have confirmed the depressant effect of anesthetics on cell growth in a variety of plants and animals. For example, Lillie (1914) determined that clinical concentrations of several inhalation anesthetics suppressed cleavage in Arbacia eggs, and that cyclopropane, chloroform, and carbon dioxide induce complete cessation of protoplasmic streaming in Mycetozoa (Seifritz, 1950).

Studies with mammalian cell cultures have further established the ability of inhalation anesthetics to reduce cell multiplication (Anderson, 1966; Fink and Kenny, 1968; Jackson, 1973; Sturrock and Nunn, 1975; Nunn, Sturrock, and Howell, 1976). Although the exact nature of this response has not been defined, it has been suggested to be associated with metaphase mitosis (Anderson, 1966) to the reversible depolymerization of mitotic spindle microtubules (Allison and Nunn, 1968) to inhibition of DNA synthesis (Bruce and Traurig, 1969; Jackson, 1973) to interference with prometaphase movement (Brinkley and Rao, 1973), or to prolongation of the G_2 postsynthetic phase (Sturrock and Nunn, 1975).

Not only have all anesthetic agents tested been shown to slow cellular division, but administration of certain anesthetics also results in production of abnormal products of mitosis (Brinkley and Rao, 1973; Sturrock and Nunn, 1975; Grant, Powell, and Radford, 1977). It has also been reported that halothane and nitrous oxide exert a synergistic action resulting in increased production of cells with abnormal nuclei (Sturrock and Nunn, 1976). The consequences of interference with the normal mitotic process in the developing organism are severe. Prolonged exposure of several animal species at critical periods of gestation to clinical concentrations of the volatile anesthetics has been shown to result in significant deformities in their offspring (Fink, Shepard, and Blandau, 1967; Basford and Fink, 1968; Smith, Gaub, and Moya, 1965; Smith, Gaub, and Lehrer, 1968; Snegireff, Cox, and Eastwood, 1968).

The effects of anesthetics on spermatogenesis are of particular interest since they exert a direct effect on the reproductive process.

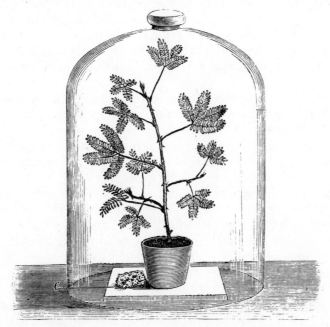

Figure 5-1 Seedlings exposed to ether vapor evidence retardation of growth. (From Bernard, Chapter 7, J.B. Balliere et Fils, 1878).

Studies in rats chronically exposed to nitrous oxide (Kripke, et al., 1976) indicate damage to the seminiferous tubules, including a reduction in sperm count and the production of abnormal multinucleated cells. Effects appear within 14 days of anesthetic administration; however, responses return to normal within a short period after cessation of the subanesthetic exposure.

Cytotoxic effects associated with the administration of nitrous oxide were demonstrated in human bone marrow by Lassen et al. (1956). These investigators noted development of granulocytopenia and thrombocytopenia in tetanus patients treated with extended inhalations of nitrous oxide. After observing the spindle destruction and chromosomal abnormalities which appeared in exposed embryonic mouse heart fibroblasts, Kieler, Mortenson, and Peterson (1957) suggested that nitrous oxide is a mitotic poison. Green and Eastwood (1963) also observed toxic effects in bone marrow cells, accompanied by a decrease in peripheral white blood count in rats chronically exposed to nitrous oxide. Similar leucopenic effects have been reported in the rat (Parbrook, 1967; Kripke et al., 1977). On the other hand, other workers have reported that intermittent exposures of rats to low concentrations of nitrous oxide (1% for six hours) resulted in only transient polycythemia without alteration in hemopoesis (Cleaton-Jones et al., 1977). Nunn et al. (1976) examined the effects of exposure to nitrous oxide, halothane, or both, on cultured rat bone marrow cells and found an inhibition of cellular growth in a dose-dependent fashion. Combination of the two anesthetics resulted in a depression of response proportional to their combined relative narcotic potencies.

Nitrous oxide has been shown to react chemically with vitamin B_{12} resulting in destruction of vitamin activity (Banks, Henderson, and Pratt, 1968). Nitrous oxide administered to patients for 6 hours produced mild, and for 24 hours, severe, signs of megaloblastic depression of the bone marrow (Amess et al., 1978). A recent report describes a specific myeloneuropathy in dentists that is associated with the abuse or prolonged occupational exposure to this anesthetic (Layzer, 1978). The neurologic picture is similar to that of subacute combined degeneration of the spinal cord, suggesting the possibility that nitrous oxide may interfere with the action of vitamin B_{12} in the nervous system.

Despite extensive in vitro and in vivo studies conducted at clinical and at subanesthetic concentration in plants, animals, and cell cultures which document the depressant effect of anesthetics on cell growth and cell division, no comparable data are available to describe the effects of long-term exposure to trace concentrations of anesthetics. In the absence of such information, we face significant difficulty in translating findings reported at clinical or subanesthetic concentration to causal effects which might apply to the low trace anesthetic concentrations present in the operating room. Nonetheless, it would seem reasonable to assume a positive relationship.

ROLE OF ANESTHETIC METABOLISM

The past decade has witnessed an explosion of interest with respect to metabolism of the volatile anesthetics. From a long-held and complacent belief as to the inertness of these agents, we have awakened to the realization that all clinically useful inhalation anesthetics are metabolized in the body. Most significant are emerging data which implicate an association between anesthetic metabolism and the development of acute and long-term toxicity. In many instances, both hypersensitivity and long-term toxicity may be explained on the basis of anesthetic metabolism. During the process of metabolism, free radicals and reactive intermediates are formed which covalently bond to tissue macromolecules. These intermediates also have the ability to form haptens, leading to the possible development of hypersensitivity-induced cellular damage.

Enzyme Induction

Induction of liver drug-metabolizing enzymes has been shown by many investigators to play an important role in the development of anesthetic toxicity. An established example of the association between increased anesthetic biodegradation and anesthetic toxicity is provided in studies of chloroform metabolism (Scholler, 1970). In these studies, rats exposed to chloroform anesthesia for 30 minutes demonstrated significant elevations in serum enzyme levels (SGOT and SGPT) with evidence of associated central-lobular liver necrosis (Figure 5-2). Animals pretreated with phenobarbital (an inducer of drug metabolism) showed marked increases in serum enzyme levels and further increases in the area of liver necrosis. On the other hand, rats pretreated with disulfiram (an inhibitor of drug-metabolizing enzymes) evidenced no increase in serum enzyme levels or in liver damage when compared to unanesthetized controls.

Similar data have been obtained for the anesthetic fluroxene. Studies conducted on several animal species associate metabolism of this inhalation anesthetic with increased levels of toxicity (Blake, Rozman, and Cascorbi, 1967; Cascorbi and Singh-Amaranath, 1972; Harrison and Smith, 1973; Johnston et al., 1973; Munson, Malagodi, and Shields, 1975). Pretreatment of the animals with phenobarbital results in increased production of the anesthetic metabolite trifluoroethanol and in an increase in mortality. Pretreatment with carbon tetrachloride or actinomycin D, on the other hand, inhibits liver enzyme activity and significantly reduces anesthetic metabolism and hepatotoxicity.

Direct evidence for an association between anesthetic metabolism and anesthetic toxicity in humans is provided by studies with methoxyflurane anesthesia. Metabolism of this anesthetic results in a significant release of inorganic fluoride. This increase in fluoride level has been shown to result in the development of nephrotoxicity in a dose-dependent fashion following prolonged methoxyflurane anesthetic administration (Taves et al., 1970; Mazze, Trudell, and Cousins, 1971).

The metabolism of halothane offers a reasonable explanation for the rare cases of hepatotoxicity which follow its administration, although this relationship has been difficult to define in humans. A recently developed more dependable animal model clearly indicates

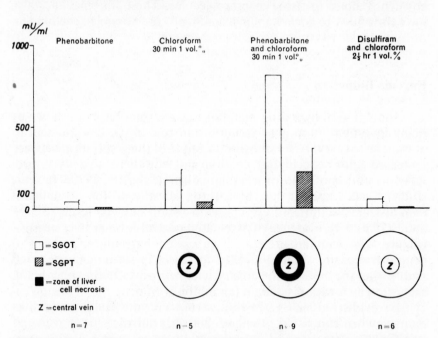

Figure 5-2 Serum enzyme levels and liver necrosis in rats 24 hours following chloroform anesthesia with and without pretreatment with phenobarbital or disulfiram. Zone of liver necrosis drawn to proportionate scale. (From Scholler, *Br J Anaesth.* 42:603–608, 1970. Reprinted by permission of the publisher Macmillian Journals Ltd. and of the author).

the presence of an association between anesthetic metabolism and anesthetic toxicity (Reynolds and Moslen, 1974; Sipes and Brown, 1976). The rat model has further demonstrated the contributory role of hypoxia in promoting reductive metabolism and an increase in halothane toxicity (Widger, Gandolfi, and Van Dyke, 1976).

Despite the fact that measured concentrations of waste anesthetic in the operating room are exceedingly low, they may be sufficient to produce measurable alterations in metabolism in the chronically exposed individual. Data furnished by Cascorbi et al. (1970) suggest an increase in halothane urinary metabolites produced by exposed anesthetists. Although a statistically significant increase was not clear from this study, other evidence indicates significant increases in drug-metabolizing enzymes following anesthetic exposure. For example, decreases in antipyrine clearance in operating room personnel have been reported (Wood et al., 1974), as well as a reduction in warfarin half-life (Ghoneim et al., 1975). Studies in animals further suggest that a higher proportionate amount of anesthetic metabolism occurs at lower anesthetic concentrations (Sawyer et al., 1971; Reynolds and Moslen, 1975). This result would favor increased biodegradation of trace concentrations of anesthetic present in the operating room. The association between increased anesthetic metabolism and increased levels of toxicity was emphasized earlier.

Excreted Metabolites

Excretion of anesthetic metabolites in the exhaled air, urine, and feces, is the normal route for elimination. Although certain anesthetic metabolites have been determined to be toxic, this toxicity usually occurs only at very high concentrations, which are infrequently reached. On the other hand, an increased level of retained anesthetic metabolite may result from induction of drug-metabolizing enzymes, or follow the decreased elimination of formed metabolites in the presence of reduced renal function.

Although the chemical characteristics for several of the excreted anesthetic metabolites have been identified, significant toxicity has been shown to exist for only a few.

Inorganic Fluoride Metabolic release of inorganic fluoride has been demonstrated for each of the clinically used fluorinated anesthetics. The extent of defluorination varies over a broad range and is dependent upon specific enzymatic defluorinase activity and the lipid solubility characteristics of the anesthetic. Considering four commonly used fluorine-containing anesthetics, the relative levels of defluorination are methoxyflurane > enflurane > isoflurane >

halothane. Levels of serum inorganic fluoride in excess of 50 $\mu M/L$ are associated with an interference in sodium transport at the proximal convoluted tubule and result in high-output renal failure (Kosek, Mazze, and Cousins, 1972; Cousins, Mazze, and Kosek, 1974). Lower serum fluoride levels presumably are less toxic.

Studies with methoxyflurane indicate a pronounced effect of phenobarbital induction on the increased production of inorganic fluoride and development of renal toxicity (Cousins et al., 1974; Adler, Brown, and Thompson, 1976). Conversely, pretreatment of the animals with the enzyme inhibitor SKF 525-A prevents attainment of toxic levels of inorganic fluoride (Berman and Bochantin, 1970; Cousins et al., 1974).

Normally, the release of inorganic fluoride from halothane is limited in amount. However, increased levels of fluoride release and increased toxicity following halothane administration occur following preanesthetic enzyme induction of the experimental animals with both phenobarbital and Aroclor 1254 (Reynolds and Moslen, 1974; Sipes and Brown, 1976). A shift toward reductive metabolism and an increased release of fluoride ion has been reported to be associated with hypoxia (Widger et al., 1976).

Inorganic Bromine Release of bromide ion following halothane anesthesia has been shown to be dose-dependent (Atallah and Geddes, 1973; Johnston et al., 1975; Tinker, Gandolfi, and Van Dyke, 1976; Duvaldestin et al., 1979). Peak bromine levels are reached by the second to sixth postoperative day and, on rare occasion, may reach psychoactive levels. No clinical data are presently available to quantify the contributory effect of enzyme induction upon bromine release, although increased levels of bromine excretion following halothane anesthesia would be expected under these circumstances.

Trifluoroacetic Acid Trifluoroacetic acid, a major urinary metabolite, has been identified in humans and in several animal species following anesthesia with halothane, fluroxene, or isoflurane. The compound, however, has proven to be of low-level toxicity when chronically administered to mice or rats in their drinking water. Ingestion results in enlargement of the liver with coordinated growth, in an increase in protein, and in an accompanying decrease in pyruvate kinase activity and glycerol 1-phosphate oxidase (Stier et al., 1972).

Trifluoroethanol The toxic metabolite trifluoroethanol is an established end product of fluroxene biodegradation and a suggested, but not proven, metabolite of halothane. Species variability in the metabolism of fluroxene favors reduced formation of this metabolite in humans, but trifluoroethanol has been demonstrated in toxic concentrations in many experimental species following its administration.

The influence of phenobarbital induction is to produce increased fluroxene metabolism and increased toxicity. This finding has been confirmed by several investigators (Blake et al., 1967; Cascorbi and Singh-Amaranath, 1973; Harrison and Smith, 1973; Munson et al., 1975). Recent studies by Harrison et al. (1976) with three anesthetic agents closely related chemically to fluroxene indicate that the trifluoroethyl moiety provides a common denominator with respect to this toxicity.

Oxalic Acid   Increased urinary excretion of oxalic acid follows methoxyflurane anesthesia, and crystalline oxalate deposits have been demonstrated in the kidneys. Although renal toxicity as a result of tubular obstruction has been shown to result from high urinary oxalate concentration, toxicity occurs only at concentrations significantly greater than those present following the clinical use of methoxyflurane. The renal lesion produced by methoxyflurane is also histologically and functionally different from that seen with oxalate (Cousins et al., 1974).

Volatile Metabolites   Several volatile metabolites of halothane have been demonstrated recently in humans. These are present in the ppm range and include trifluorochloroethane, difluorochloroethylene, and difluorobromochloroethylene (Sharp, Trudell, and Cohen, 1979). The latter compound is of potential concern in that its LC_{50} in rats is only 250 ppm (Raventos and Lemon, 1965). Not only is this substance produced biologically in the body as a result of halothane metabolism, but increased amounts are generated during closed-circuit anesthesia as a result of a chemical interaction of halothane with soda lime (Sharp, et al., 1978). The Ames test for mutagenicity is positive for this metabolite, as well as for difluorochloroethylene (Edmunds, Baden, and Simmons, in press). Although the possibility of clinical toxicity must be considered, no relevant data exist in humans.

REACTIVE INTERMEDIATES

The halogenated inhalation anesthetic agents were previously considered to be nonreactive, but it now appears that under appropriate conditions, they are metabolized to reactive intermediates or free radicals capable of combining with cellular constituents. There are a number of ways in which free radicals might be produced by metabolism of an anesthetic drug. For example, hydroxylation and dehalogenation of halothane by its interaction with the cytochrome P_{450} system could produce a reactive acyl halide:

$$\underset{\substack{| \ | \\ F \ Cl}}{\overset{\substack{F \ Br \\ | \ |}}{F-C-C-H}} \quad \xrightarrow{P_{450}} \quad \underset{\substack{| \\ F-Cl}}{\overset{\substack{F \ Br \\ | \ |}}{F-C-C-OH}} \quad \xrightarrow{-HBr} \quad \underset{\substack{| \\ F}}{\overset{\substack{F \ O \\ | \ ||}}{F-C-C-Cl}}$$

It has also been suggested that, under certain conditions, cytochrome P_{450} is capable of removing a proton to form a reactive carbanion (Ullrich and Schnabel, 1973):

$$\underset{\substack{| \ | \\ F \ Cl}}{\overset{\substack{F \ Br \\ | \ |}}{F-C-C-H}} \quad \xrightarrow{-H^{+}} \quad \underset{\substack{| \ | \\ F \ Cl}}{\overset{\substack{F \ Br \\ | \ |}}{F-C-C^{\cdot}}}$$

By analogy, with the work of Van Duuren and his colleagues (1972) on the alpha-haloethers, it is possible that the following reaction may also occur:

$$\underset{\substack{| \ | \\ F \ Cl}}{\overset{\substack{F \ Br \\ | \ |}}{F-C-C-H}} \quad \xrightarrow{-Br} \quad \underset{\substack{| \ | \\ F \ Cl}}{\overset{\substack{F \ H \\ | \ |}}{F-C-C^{\cdot}}}$$

Formation of free radicals and reactive intermediates is consistent with evidence showing that the metabolites bind covalently to liver microsomes and to tissue macromolecules.

Cellular damage produced as a result of binding of a reactive metabolite may vary depending on the molecular aggregate formed. Molecules with the highest susceptibility for damage include the unsaturated fatty acids and nucleic acids. Fatty acid complexes of phosphatidylcholine and phosphatidylethanolamine form the major membrane components of liver endoplasmic reticulum and mitochondria. Since inhalation anesthetic agents are strongly lipophilic, they can be expected to be closely associated with these lipoprotein membranes. The lipid constituents are particularly rich in unsaturated fatty acids, and binding of the reactive intermediates would tend to occur within this milieu (Figure 5-3).

Brown (1972) provided evidence of hepatic microsomal lipoperoxidation in the rat following administration of chloroform and halothane. Using rats pretreated with phenobarbital, he measured the increase in diene conjugation in hepatic microsomes resulting from lipoperoxidation. Brown, Sipes, and Sagalyn (1974) also found that in animals pretreated with phenobarbital, chloroform anesthesia produced a decrease in the liver content of glutathione and an increase in hepatic necrosis. Pretreatment with diethyl malate decreased glutathione concentration and was associated with liver damage. It appears that if the tissue concentrations of these antioxidants reach critically low values, the reactive metabolites formed from chloroform are no longer quenched and become free to promote tissue damage by lipoperoxidation.

Evidence for the covalent binding of reactive halothane metabolites to tissue macromolecules comes from several sources (Uehleke, Hellmer, and Tarbelli-Poplawski, 1973; Van Dyke and Wood, 1973; Van Dyke and Gandolfi, 1974). Additional experiments also indicate a threefold increase in binding to microsomal lipids in hypoxic rats which is associated with a significant increase in serum inorganic fluoride (Widger et al., 1976).

Also of significant concern are studies which indicate covalent binding of halothane metabolites to macromolecules within the liver. These reactive intermediates are able to bind to both lipids and proteins. Gandolfi and Van Dyke (In press) showed that the binding of phospholipids is through the fatty acid moiety. Highest lipid binding occurs in the phospholipid fraction, most specifically to phosphatidylethanolamine. This binding is enhanced at lower oxygen tension, following diethyl malate-induced glutathione depletion or

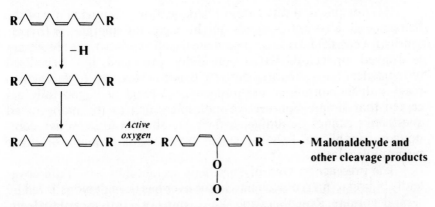

Figure 5-3 Possible mechanism for lipoperoxidation. (From Brown, *Anesthesiology.* 36:458–465, 1972. Reprinted by permission of the publisher J.B. Lippincott, and of the author.)

after pretreatment of the animal with a diet rich in polyunsaturated fatty acids. Enzyme induction increases production of reactive intermediates and tends to promote increased binding. Hypoxia and reduced antioxidant concentration act to prolong the half-life of the intermediates and result in increased binding.

Although significant covalent binding of metabolites also occurs to liver proteins, the identities of the metabolites and specific binding sites to individual proteins or amino acids are not known. It would also appear that the binding to DNA and RNA is limited, although measurable binding may occur to chromatin and to ribosomal protein (Edmunds et al., in press). These observations are of potential interest in terms of possible interference with the genetic process, but their significance remains to be determined.

The metabolic pathways described indicate that biodegradation of halothane may proceed along both oxidative and reductive routes. Under aerobic conditions, metabolism preferentially leads to fluoride, bromide, and trifluoroacetic acid. Widger, et al. (1976) investigated the effects of reduced oxygen tension on the metabolism of halothane. Rats exposed to a 7% inhaled oxygen concentration responded with significantly increased concentrations of fluoride ions in their plasma. This increase in dehalogenation under hypoxic conditions was also accompanied by a more than threefold increase in the covalent binding of metabolites to the microsomal lipids. This greater binding during hypoxia supports the hypothesis that reductive metabolism produces a more reactive chemical species.

HYPERSENSITIVITY AND THE IMMUNE RESPONSE

It is possible that rare cases of hepatic injury following use of the halogenated anesthetic agents might have an allergic or hypersensitivity basis. The reactions seen are usually considered to represent a delayed or cell-mediated sensitivity produced by specialized mononuclear cells, thymus-derived lymphocytes, or T cells which react with membrane-bound antigens. Although it is generally accepted that simple nonreactive molecules such as the halogenated anesthetics cannot be antigens, their metabolites are reactive compounds capable of forming stable bonds with proteins or other macromolecules.

The presence in vivo of anesthetic metabolites which are covalently bound to macromolecules in the liver has been demonstrated by several workers. Rosenberg and Wahlstrom (1973) attempted to determine if trifluoroacetic acid and other "presumed" halothane metabolites could act as haptens in the rabbit. Although their results suggest that the immune serum formed similar precipitins against these complexes, the evidence is not totally convincing. Later studies by Mathieu et al. (1974) using a trifluoroacetyl guinea pig albumin complex showed that guinea pigs displayed a typical delayed-type hypersensitivity. The fact that a delayed skin hypersensitivity can be induced, however, does not mean that such hapten complexes are also capable of causing autoimmune liver destruction.

The presence of a previous exposure to halothane in more than half the reported cases of hepatitis is in accord with the widely held sensitization hypothesis. However, with the prevalent use of this anesthetic, multiple exposures would be expected to occur with increasing frequency. A small number of individuals with previous episodes of hepatitis have actually undergone challenge tests with halothane (Belfrage, Ahlgren, and Axelsom, 1966; Klatskin and Kimberg, 1969). These two well-known cases where anesthetists were challenged with small doses of halothane attest to the existence of hypersensitivity reaction, although the validity of these reports has been questioned (Simpson, Strunin, and Walton, 1973). Finally, there are data which suggest a significant relationship between repeated exposures to halothane and the rapidity with which jaundice develops following subsequent exposure (Inman and Mushin, 1974). Although there appears to be a decreasing time interval for the development of jaundice following repeated exposure to halothane, these data have also come under question. Thus, while it is tempting to postulate a causal relationship between the hypersensitivity response and hepatotoxicity of halothane, the data are not secure.

SAFE LEVELS OF OCCUPATIONAL ANESTHETIC EXPOSURE

Although many published reports strongly suggest the presence of an occupational hazard in the operating room presumably associated with the waste anesthetic gases, "safe levels of chronic anesthetic inhalation" have not been established. The recently published NIOSH Criteria Document suggests an acceptable exposure level of 2 ppm for halogenated anesthetics and 25 ppm for nitrous oxide. In the absence of precise biologic data, such limits are based on the lowest concentrations of anesthetic detectable or reasonably attainable. Varying standards have been established in other countries. For example, the Hospital Engineering Cooperative Group of Denmark (1974) has recommended lower exposure levels than those suggested by NIOSH. Permissible average concentrations in the breathing zone of anesthesia personnel were set at 1 ppm for halothane, 10 ppm for nitrous oxide, and intermediate levels for other anesthetics. The Swedish Labor Protection Board (1975), while not establishing environmental levels, suggested that operating rooms be required to have 17 air exchanges per hour and that gases flowing out of valves on the anesthesia equipment be carried away from the work area.

A recent study (Halsey, 1978) attempted to combine data from several human and animal sources in an effort to estimate minimum threshold anesthetic concentrations producing significant effects on fertility, spontaneous abortion, fetal retardation, and fetal abnormality, pathological organ changes, carcinogenicity, mutagenicity, or performance impairment. The limiting factors varied significantly for each agent, but after allowing a threefold safety factor, the author suggested the following maximum safe levels of anesthetic contamination: nitrous oxide–330 ppm; trichloroethylene–100 ppm; enflurane–20 ppm; halothane–5 ppm; methoxyflurane–5 ppm. These concentrations refer to time-averaged exposures and are based on both animal and human data. They assume individual exposures of less than 12 hours daily. Since the anesthetic levels suggested exceed those at which health hazards have been reported in humans, the applicability of these combined data to the clinical situation may be questioned. In addition, in clinical practice, more than one inhalation anesthetic agent is usually present, and in combination, these agents may act with an additive effect with regard to overall toxicity.

Another estimate of "safe" concentration levels may be obtained by examining the incidence of health responses in those professional groups working in the operating room at different levels of anesthetic exposure. Thus, the physician anesthetists may be in the operating room for longer periods than the nurse anesthetist, whereas the operating room nurse or technician is exposed to anesthetic concentrations significantly less than the anesthetist. Data obtained from the national ASA study (Cohen et al., 1974) suggest that female physician anesthetists have higher rates of liver disease and cancer than nurse anesthetists. Both rates, in turn, are significantly higher than those for operating room nurses or technicians who work at greater distance from the source of anesthetic gases. The data on reproductive hazard, however, prove inconsistent in defining a dose-response relationship. "Safe" concentration levels must therefore be interpreted with caution, and it would seem most prudent to attempt to maintain anesthetic concentrations in the room at their lowest reasonably attainable level.

NONANESTHETIC HAZARDS IN THE OPERATING ROOM

Although waste anesthetics offer obvious intrusion to the air quality of the operating room, there are a number of additional physical and chemical contaminants that are also present. These include ultraviolet and x-radiation, freon gases used as propellants, halogenated hydrocarbons applied as defatting agents, volatile by-products generated during the preparation of surgical cement, etc. In addition the operating room must be regarded as a milieu of high emotional stress. It may be argued that any or all of these additional factors can produce health effects upon personnel exposed to their influences.

X-Ray Ultraviolet, and Radiofrequency Energies

The toxic effects of x-radiation are well known, and current federal regulations assign safe exposure levels at 100 milliroentgens per week (Code of Federal Regulations, Title 10, 1972). An earlier study has determined the level of x-ray exposure in anesthetists during the course of usual operating room activities over a six-week period (Linde and Bruce, 1969). Although mean exposure averaged only 13 milliroentgens per week, wide variation was noted in individual anesthetists. In addition, the average weekly exposure level dropped significantly after the first week, suggesting increased awareness by the anesthetist associated with the wearing of a dosimeter. It would thus appear that although the anesthetist may at times be inadvertantly exposed to an undesirable level of radiation, the risk is small, and permanent injuries have not been reported (Williamson, Parks, and Samsen, 1972; Martinenghi et al., 1977).

It is of interest to consider the possible combined toxic effects that may exist between exposure to anesthetics plus x-radiation. Although human data are not available, such an interaction has been described in mice (Bruce and Koepke, 1969); unfortunately, it is not presently clear whether the effects are protective (Evans, Roberts, and Orkin, 1964) or potentiating (Schultz, Markoe, and Anigstein, 1969). An additional concern would appear to be associated with the destructive effect of ionizing radiation on the anesthetic itself. In the case of halothane, exposure of the anesthetic to x-radiation results in formation of significant amounts of the toxic decomposition product dichlorohexafluorobutene (Pennington, 1968). Exposure of nitrous oxide to ionizing radiation leads to formation of toxic higher oxides of nitrogen, including nitric oxide and nitrogen dioxide (Goldstein et al., 1976).

Other sources of energy release are also to be found in the operating room. These include use of electrocautery, cardiac defibrillators, laser beams, and ultraviolet radiation. The released energies of the electrocautery have been determined by radio-frequency (RF) equipment, and power flux densities in excess of 150 mW/cm^2 have been reported at the point of application of the Bovie probe (Fox, Knadle, and Brook, 1976). Chemiluminescent monitors indicate that nitrous oxide levels of 0.6 ppm and nitrogen dioxide levels of 0.15 ppm may also be present during intensive use of these devices (Goldstein et al., 1976). Fortunately, measured levels for the higher oxides of nitrogen are below American Industrial Hygiene limits of 25 ppm for nitric oxide and 5 ppm for nitrogen dioxide.

A fetal damaging effect of electromagnetic irradiation on pregnant female mice has been demonstrated following four minutes of exposure to a 7.3-W microwave waveguide at 2450 MHz (Hugh and McManawy, 1976). In this instance, the addition of pentobarbital anesthesia to the mother protected the fetus, presumably by immobilization of the mother, plus a further action of the anesthetic in reducing body temperature (–4 to 5 °C). The former effect served to limit the area of microwave exposure, and the cooling effect compensated for the thermal damaging effects of the microwave radiation.

Ultraviolet light has been used in operating rooms for the control of infection. Experimental studies indicate decomposition of halothane following its exposure to ultraviolet light, which acts to release free fluoride ion and the formation of unknown toxic decomposition product(s) (Karis et al., 1976). Mice exposed to ultraviolet-irradiated halothane lost weight and developed hemorrhagic lesions in the lung and vacuolization of the liver. These findings were absent in animals exposed to the nonirradiated halothane.

Freon Propellants

Freon gases have been used to provide the propellant force in many areosol sprays used for dressing surgical wounds. The most common of these freon gases are dichlorofluoromethane (freon 12) and trichlorofluoromethane (freon 13). It has been demonstrated in dogs that fluorocarbon levels as low as 20 to 35 μg/ml may sensitize the heart to arrhythmias (Jack, 1971). Since many of the anesthetics are also myocardial irritants, it has been suggested that a summation effect might occur in individuals simultaneously exposed to freons plus the waste anesthetic gases (Hunter, 1976).

Methylmethacrylate

The use of self-curing plastic surgical cement has permitted important advances in orthopedic and reconstructive facial surgery. Unfortunately, release of the toxic monomer, methylmethacrylate, occurs during mixing and setting stages of the cement. Reported toxic effects include hypotension, occasional cardiac arrest, and patient death (Burgess, Gresham, and Kuczynski, 1970; Power et al., 1970; Cohen and Smith, 1971). During the mixing stages, there is significant release of monomer to the room air which exposes the surgeon, scrub nurse, and anesthetists to toxic vapors. Symptoms of headache, nausea, gastrointestinal upset, and abnormal liver enzymes have been noted (Milliken, Milliken, and Marshall, 1976). The LC_{50} of methylmethacrylate monomer inhalation in the rat has been established at 13,500 ppm following a 3-hour exposure (Fassett, 1967). Measurements of methylmethacrylate concentration present in the operating room during total hip procedures indicate peak concentrations of 227 ppm during the first few minutes of cement mixing, followed by a rapid fall off to < 10 ppm within 11 minutes (McLaughlin et al., 1978). Fortunately, these concentrations are below OSHA-established exposure standards of 100 ppm over a period of 8 hours (FDA Regulations, 1966). Teratogenicity and fetal toxicity studies in the pregnant mouse indicate no significant toxicity upon exposure to methylmethacrylate vapor levels as high as 1300 ppm for two hours twice daily during day 6 through day 15 of gestation (McLaughlin et al., 1978). Thus, although toxicity from methylmethacrylate inhalation cannot be excluded, significant clinical hazard associated with the surgical use of cements remains to be determined.

Stress and the Operating Room

Although relatively few physicians view the operating room as the critical center of hospital activity, most agree that this area does represent a focus of significant emotional stress. Physicians and nurses working in the operating room are considered to be subject to high levels of continuous pressure. It is perhaps no wonder that the suicide rate, high among physicians, is even higher among anesthetists (Bruce et al., 1968). Further, it seems reasonable to consider operating room stress as a possible contributory cause of increased health risks observed among surgical and anesthesia personnel.

Emotion and stress are known to influence essential physiologic mechanisms and have been implicated as contributory to numerous health problems, including birth defects, miscarriages, and cancer. Responses originating within the central nervous system are mediated through the neuroendocrine system. Serum corticosteroids play an important role and are shown to increase during stress. Stress and elevated serum steroid levels have been reported to be assocated with abnormal fetal osteogenesis in the mouse (Barlow et al., 1974). Catecholamines are likewise involved, and plasma norepinephrine levels have been shown to increase significantly in operating theater personnel on operating days (Mehta and Burton, 1976). On the other hand, plasma cortisol and urinary adrenaline levels remain unchanged (Mehta and Burton, 1977).

A number of studies appear to offer positive correlation between occupational stress and the risk of disease. Workers at management level have been shown to be subject to greater stress than their employees and as a consequence suffer an increased incidence of hypertension, heart disease, obesity, and duodenal ulcer (Weiman, 1977). Women who habitually abort (three or more consecutive spontaneous abortions) have shown frequent emotional instability, evidenced by poor emotional content, stronger dependency needs, and greater anxiety than their control group (Grimm, 1962; Mann, 1957, McDonald, 1968).

Studies investigating mental retardation in children also suggest close association between illness and stress of the mother during pregnancy and outcome of the pregnancy (Stott, 1957). Other studies demonstrate an association between cleft palate and stress reactions experienced around the sixtieth day of pregnancy. In 228 cases of cleft palate, 85% of the mothers reported stressful episodes during this period (Strean and Peer, 1958). A more recent study indicates a positive correlation between the effects of anxiety during the first trimester and an increase in abnormalities of pregnancy and infant status (Gorsch and Key, 1974).

Although the data are limited, several studies have suggested an association between emotional stress and the pathogenesis of cancer in humans (LeShan, 1959; Taylor, 1974). It has also been suggested that a positive correlation exists between psychological factors and the growth rate of human cancer (Blumberg, West, and Ellis, 1954). In this study, the Minnesota Multiphasic Personality Inventory (MMPI) was administered to a series of 50 cancer patients. Striking differences in test results were obtained between two groups of patients with respect to disease activity and length of survival. It was considered that development of cancer in humans could conceivably result from the physiologic effects of long-continued inner stress which remained unresolved by either outward action or successful adaptation. The authors concluded that cancer may represent a nonadaptation syndrome.

On the basis of the preceding studies, it remains possible that operating room stress plays a positive role in the increased health risks noted in operating room personnel. At the present time, however, data are insufficient to define the true significance of this possibility. Further studies are urgently needed. In the meantime, we believe there is significant evidence to suggest that anesthetic waste gases in the operating room offer the most reasonable explanation for the increased health hazards noted in operating room personnel.

REFERENCES

Adler, L., Brown, B.R., and Thompson, M.F. Kinetics of methoxyflurane biotransformation with reference to substrate inhibition. *Anesthesiology.* 44:380–385, 1976.

Allison, A.C., and Nunn, J.F. Effects of general anesthetics on micro-tubules: A possible mechanism of anesthesia. *Lancet.* 2:1396–1329, 1968.

Amess, J., Burman, J., Rees, G., et al. Megaloblastic haemopoiesis in patients receiving nitrous oxide. *Lancet.* 2:339–342, 1978.

Anderson, N.B. The effects of CNS depressants on mitosis. *Acta Anaesthesiol Scand.* 22:(suppl) 1–36, 1966.

Atallah, M.M., and Geddes, I.C. Metabolism of halothane during and after anesthesia in man. *Br J Anaesth.* 45:464–469, 1973.

Banks, R., Henderson, R., and Pratt, J. Reactions of gases in solution. III. Some reactions of nitrous oxide with transition-metal complexes. *J Chem Soc.* Sec 12 (A), 2886, 1968.

Barlow, S., McElhatton, P., Morrison, P., et al. Effects of stress during pregnancy on plasma corticosterone levels and foetal development in the mouse. *J Physiol (Lond).* 239:35–56, 1974.

Basford, A., and Fink, B.R. Teratogenic activity of halothane in rats. *Anesthesiology.* 29:1167–1173, 1968.

Belfrage, S., Ahlgren, I., and Axelson, I. Halothane hepatitis in an anaesthetist. *Lancet.* 2:1466–1467, 1966.

Berman, M.L., and Bochantin, B.S. Nonspecific stimulation of drug metabolism in rats by methoxyflurane. *Anesthesiology.* 32:500–506, 1970.

Bernard, C. Leçon sur les phenomenes de la vie communns aux animaux et aux vegetaux. 7, Paris: J.B. Balliere et Fils, 1878.

Blake, D.A., Rozman, R.S., and Cascorbi, H.F. Anesthesia LX-XIV: Biotransformation of fluroxene. I. Metabolism in mice and dogs in vivo. *Biochem Pharmacol.* 16:1237–1248, 1967.

Blumberg, E.M., West, P.M., and Ellis, F.W. A possible relationship between psychological factors and human cancer. *Psychosom Med.* 16:227–286, 1954.

Brinkley, B.R., and Rao, P.N. Nitrous oxide: Effects on the mitotic apparatus and chromosome movement in HeLa cells. *J Cell Biol.* 58:96–106, 1973.

Brown, B.R. Hepatic microsomal lipoperoxidation and inhalation anesthetics: A biochemical and morphologic study in the rat. *Anesthesiology.* 36:458–465, 1972.

Brown, B.R., and Sagalyn, A.M. Hepatic microsomal enzyme induction by inhalation anesthetics. *Anesthesiology.* 40:152–161, 1974.

Brown, B.R., Sipes, I.G., and Sagalyn, A.M. Mechanisms of acute hepatic toxicity: Chloroform, halothane, and glutathione. *Anesthesiology.* 41:554–561, 1974.

Bruce, D.L., Eide, K.A., Linde, H.W., et al. Causes of death among anesthesiologists: A 20-year survey. *Anesthesiology.* 29:565–569, 1968.

Bruce, D.L., and Traurig, H. The effect of halothane on the cell cycle in rat small intestine. *Anesthesiology.* 30:401–405, 1969.

Bruce, D.L., and Koepke, J.A. Interaction of halothane and radiation in mice: Possible implications. *Anesth Analg (Cleve).* 48:687–694, 1969.

Burgess, D.M. Gresham, G.A., and Kuczynski, A. Cardiac arrest and bone cement. *Br Med J.* 3:465, 1970.

Cascorbi, H.F., Blake, D.A., and Helrich, M. Differences in the biotransformation of halothane in man. *Anesthesiology.* 32: 119–123, 1970.

Cascorbi, H.F., and Singh-Amaranath, A.V. Modification of fluroxene toxicity. *Anesthesiology.* 38:454–457, 1973.

Clarke, D.G., and Tinston, D.J. Cardiac effects of isoproterenol, hypoxia, hypercapnia, and fluorocarbon propellants and their use in asthma inhalers. *Ann Allergy.* 30:536–541, 1972.

Cleaton-Jones, P., Austin, J.C., Banks, D., et al. Effect of intermittent exposure to a low concentration of nitrous oxide on haemopoiesis in rats. *Br J Anesth.* 49:223–226, 1977.

Code of Federal Regulations. Title 10, Part 20. Washington, D.C.: U.S. Government Printing Office, 1972.

Cohen, C.A., and Smith, T.C. The intraoperative hazard of acrylic bone cement: Report of a case. *Anesthesiology.* 35:547–549, 1971.

Cohen, E.N., Brown, B.W., Bruce, D.L., et al. Occupational disease among operating room personnel: A national study. *Anesthesiology.* 41:321–340, 1974.

Cousins, M.J., Mazze, R.I., and Kosek, J. The etiology of methoxyflurane nephrotoxicity. *J Pharmacol Exp Ther.* 190:530–541, 1974.

Duvaldestin, P., Mazze, R.I., Hazebrouck, J., et al. Halothane biotransformation in anesthetists. *Anesthesiology.* (In press)

Edmunds, H.N., Baden, J.M., and Simmon, V.F. Mutagenicity studies with volatile metabolites of halothane in man. *Anesthesiology.* (In press)

Evans, J.C., Roberts, T.W., and Orkin, L.R. Modification of radiosensitivity of mice by inert gases and nitrous oxide. *Radiat Res.* 21:243–255, 1964.

Fassett, D.W., Esters. Edited by F.A. Patty. In *Industrial Hygiene and Toxicology.* Vol II. New York: Interscience, 1967.

Fink, B.R., Shepard, T.H., and Blandau, R.J. Teratogenic activity of N_2O. *Nature.* 214:146–148, 1967.

Fink, B.R., and Kenny, G.E. Metabolic effects of volatile anesthetics in cell culture. *Anesthesiology.* 29:505–516, 1968.

Fink, B.R., and Cullen, B.F. Anesthetic pollution: What is happening to us? *Anesthesiology.* 45:79–83, 1976.

Fox, J., Knadle, R., and Brook, R. Radiofrequency in the operating theatre. *Lancet.* 1:962, 1976.

Gandolfi, A.J., and Van Dyke, R.A. Effects of animal pretreatment on the in vivo covalent binding of halothane metabolites to hepatic lipids and proteins. *Chem Biol Interact.* (In press)

Goldstein, B.D., Paz, J., Guiffrida, J.G., et al. Atmospheric derivatives of anaesthetic gases as a possible hazard to operating room personnel. *Lancet.* 2:235–236, 1976.

Ghoneim, M.M., Delle, M., Wilson, W.R., et al. Alteration of warfarin kinetics in man associated with exposure to an operating room environment. *Anesthesiology.* 43:333–336, 1975.

Gorsch, R.L., and Key, M.K. Abnormalities of pregnancy as a function of anxiety and life stress. *Psychosom Med.* 36:352–362, 1974.

Grant, G.J., Powell, J.N., and Radford, S.G. Induction of chromosomal abnormalities by inhalation anesthetics. *Mutat Res.* 46:177–184, 1977.

Green, C.D., and Eastwood, D.W. Effects of nitrous oxide inhalation on hemopoiesis in rats. *Anesthesiology.* 24:341–345, 1963.

Grimm, E. Psychological investigation of habitual abortion. *Psychosom Med.* 24:369–378, 1962.

112

Halsey, M.J. Maximum safe levels of anaesthetic contamination in operating rooms. *Br J Anaesth.* 50:633, 1978.

Harrison, G.G., and Smith, J.S. Massive lethal hepatic necrosis in rats anesthetized with fluroxene, after microsomal enzyme induction. *Anesthesiology.* 39:619–625, 1973.

Harrison, G.G., Ivanetich, K.M., Kaminsky, L., et al. Fluroxene (2, 2, 2-trifluoroethyl vinyl ether) toxicity: A chemical aspect. *Anesth Analg (Cleve).* 55:529–533, 1976.

Hugh, R., and McManawy, M. Anesthesia as an effective agent against the production of congenital anomalies in mouse fetuses exposed to electromagnetic radiation. *J Exp Zool.* 197:363–368, 1976.

Hunter, L. An occupational health approach to anaesthetic air pollution. *Med J Aust.* 1:465–468, 1976.

Inman, W.H.W., and Mushin, W.W. Jaundice after repeated exposure to halothane: An analysis of reports to the Committee on Safety of Medication. *Br Med J.* 1:5–10, 1974.

Jack, D. Sniffing syndrome. *Br Med J.* 2:708–709, 1971.

Jackson, S.H. The metabolic effects of halothane on mammalian hepatoma cells in vitro. II. Inhibition of DNA synthesis. *Anesthesiology.* 39:405–409, 1973.

Johnston, R.R., Cromwell, T.H., Eger, E.I., et al. The toxicity of fluroxene in animals and man. *Anesthesiology.* 38:313–319, 1973.

Johnstone, R.E., Kennell, E.M., Behar, M.G., et al. Increased serum bromide concentration after halothane anesthesia in man. *Anesthesiology.* 42:598–601, 1975.

Karis, J.H., Menzel, D.B., Donia, A., et al. Increase of halothane toxicity by ultraviolet irradiation. Abstracts of Scientific Papers, 1976 Annual Meeting of the American Society of Anesthesiologists, San Francisco, 1976, pp. 93–94.

Kieler, J., Mortensen, H., and Petersen, C.R. The cytologic effect of nitrous oxide at different oxygen tensions. *Acta Pharmacol Toxicol.* 13:301–308, 1957.

Klatskin, G., and Kimberg, D.V. Recurrent hepatitis attributable to halothane sensitization in anesthetists. *N Engl J Med.* 280:515–522, 1969.

Kosek, J.C., Mazze, R.I., and Cousins, M.J. The morphology and pathogenesis of nephrotoxicity following methoxyflurane (Penthrane) anesthesia: An experimental model in rats. *Lab Invest.* 27:575–580, 1972.

Kripke, B.J., Kelman, A.D., Shah, N.K., et al. Testicular reaction to prolonged exposure to nitrous oxide. *Anesthesiology.* 44:104–113, 1976.

Kripke, B.J., Talarico, L., Shah, N.K., et al. Hematologic reaction to prolonged exposure to nitrous oxide. *Anesthesiology.* 47:342–348, 1977.

Labor Protection Board. Narcosis specification for the protection of personnel against health risks through exposure to gaseous anesthetics in patient care work. No. 102. Stockholm, Sweden, February 1975.

Lassen, H.C.A., Henriksen, E., Neukirch, F., et al. Treatment of tetanus: Severe bone marrow depression after prolonged nitrous oxide anesthesia. *Lancet.* 1:527–530, 1956.

Layzer, R.B. Myeloneuropathy after prolonged exposure to nitrous oxide. *Lancet.* 2:1227–1230, 1978.

LeShan, L. Psychological states as factors in the development of malignant disease: A critical review. *J Natl Cancer Inst.* 22:1–18, 1959.

Lillie, R.S. The action of various anesthetics in suppressing cell division in sea urchin eggs. *J Biol Chem.* 17:121–140, 1914.

Linde, H.W., and Bruce, D.L. Occupational exposure of anesthetists to halothane, nitrous oxide, and radiation. *Anesthesiology.* 30:363–368, 1969.

Mann, E.C. The role of emotional determinants in habitual abortion. *Surg Clin North Am.* 37:447–458, 1957.

Martinenghi, C., Conte, L., Inversini, G., et al. Evaluation of the risk to anesthetists exposed to ionizing radiation in the hospital environment. *Health Phys.* 33:274, 1977.

Mathieu, A., Di Padua, D., Mills, J., et al. Experimental immunity to a metabolite of halothane and fluroxene: Cutaneous delayed-type hypersensitivity. *Anesthesiology.* 40:385–390, 1974.

Mazze, R.I., Trudell, J.R., and Cousins, M.J. Methoxyflurane metabolism and renal dysfunction: Clinical correlation in man. *Anesthesiology.* 35:247–252, 1971.

Mazze, R.I., Hitt, B.A., and Cousins, M.J. Effects of enzyme induction with phenobarbital on the in vivo and in vitro defluorination of isoflurane and methoxyflurane. *J Pharmacol Exp Ther.* 190:523–529, 1974.

McDonald, R.L. The role of emotional factors in obstetric complications: A review. *Psychosom Med.* 30:222–237, 1968.

McLaughlin, R.E., Roger, S.I., Barkalow, B.S., et al. Methylmethacrylate: A study of teratogenicity and fetal toxicity of the vapor in the mouse. *J Bone Joint Surg [Am.]* 60:355–358, 1978.

Mehta, S., and Burton, P. Pollution in our operating theatres. *Lancet.* 1:695, 1976.

_____. Stress in operating theatre personnel. *Anaesthesia.* 32:924–925, 1977.

Milliken, R.A., Milliken, G.M., and Marshall, B.J. OR pollution can have adverse effect on safety. *Hospitals.* 50:97–104, 1976.

Munson, E.S., Malagodi, M.H., and Shields, R.P. Fluroxene toxicity induced by phenobarbital. *Clin Pharmacol Ther.* 18:687–699, 1975.

Nunn, J.F., Sturrock, J.E., and Howell, A. Effect of inhalation anaesthetics on division of bone-marrow cells in vitro. *Br J Anaesth.* 48:75–81, 1976.

Parbrook, G.D. Leucopenic effects of prolonged nitrous oxide treatment. *Br J Anaesth.* 39:119–127, 1967.

Pennington, S.N. The effects of gamma radiation on halothane. *Anesthesiology.* 29:153–154, 1968.

Powell, J.N., McGrath, P.J., Lahiri, S.K., et al. Cardiac arrest associated with bone cement. *Br Med J.* 3:326, 1970.

Raventos, J., and Lemon, P.G. The impurities in Fluothane: Their biological properties. *Br J Anaesth.* 37:716–737, 1965.

Recknagel, R.V., and Ghoshal, A.K. Lipoperoxidation as a vector in carbon tetrachloride hepatotoxicity. *Lab Invest.* 15:132–148, 1966.

Reynolds, E.S., and Moslen, M.T. Liver injury following halothane anesthesia in phenobarbital-pretreated rats. *Biochem Pharmacol.* 23:189–195, 1974.

_____. Metabolism of (^{14}C-1) halothane in vivo: Effects of multiple halothane anesthesia, phenobarbital and carbon tetrachloride pretreatment. *Biochem Pharmacol.* 24:2075–2081, 1975.

Rietbrock, I., Lazarus, G., and Otterbein, A. Effect of halothane on the hepatic drug metabolizing system. *Naunyn Schmiedebergs Arch Pharmacol.* 273:422–426, 1972.

Rosenberg, P., and Wahlstrom, T. Trifluoroacetic acid and some possible intermediate metabolites of halothane as haptens. *Anesthesiology.* 38:224–227, 1973.

Sawyer, D.C., Eger, E.I., Bahlman, S.H., et al. Concentration dependence of hepatic halothane metabolism. *Anesthesiology.* 34:230–234, 1971.

Scholler, K.L. Modification of the effects of chloroform on the rat liver. *Br J Anaesth.* 42:603–605, 1970.

Schultz, R.J., Markoe, A.M., and Anigstein, R. Xenon: Effect on radiation sensitivity of HeLa cells. *Science.* 163:571–572, 1969.

Seifriz, W. The effects of various anesthetic agents on protoplasm. *Anesthesiology.* 11:24–32, 1950.

Sharp, H., Trudell, J.R., and Cohen, E.N. Volatile metabolites and decomposition products of halothane in man. *Anesthesiology.* 50:2-8, 1979.

Simpson, B.R. Strunin, L., and Walton, B. Halothane hepatitis: Fact or fallacy? *Acta Anaesthesiol Belg.* 2:133-146, 1973.

Sipes, I.G., and Brown, B.R. An animal model of hepatotoxicity associated with halothane anesthesia. *Anesthesiology.* 45:622-628, 1976.

Smith, B.E., Gaub, M.L., and Moya, F. Investigation into the teratogenic effects of anesthetic agents. *Anesthesiology.* 26:260-261, 1965.

Smith B.E., Gaub, M.L., and Lehrer, S.B. Teratogenic effects of diethyl ether in the chick embyro. Edited by B.R. Fink. In *Toxicity of Anesthetics.* Baltimore, Maryland: Williams and Wilkins Co., 1968.

Snegireff, S.L., Cox, J.R., and Eastwood, D.W. The effect of N_2O, cyclopropane, or halothane on neural tube mitotic index, weight, mortality, and growth anomaly rate in the developing chick embryo. Edited by B.R. Fink. In *Toxicity of Anesthetics.* Baltimore, Maryland: Williams and Wilkins Co., 1968.

Stevens, W.C., Eger, E.I., White, A., et al. Comparative toxicities of halothane, isoflurane, and diethyl ether at subanesthetic concentrations in laboratory animals. *Anesthesiology.* 42:408-419, 1975.

Stier, A., Kunz, W.H., Walli, A.K., et al. Effects on growth and metabolism of rat liver by halothane and its metabolite, trifluoroacetate. *Biochem Pharmacol.* 21:2181-2192, 1972.

Stott, D.H. Psychophysical and mental handicaps following a disturbed pregnancy. *Lancet.* 1:1006-1011, 1957.

Strean, L.P., and Peer, L.A. Stress as an etiologic factor in the development of cleft palate. *Plast Reconstr Surg.* 18:1-8, 1958.

Sturrock, J.E., and Nunn, J.F. Mitosis in mammalian cells during exposure to anesthetics. *Anesthesiology.* 43:21-33, 1975.

_____. Effects of halothane on DNA synthesis and the presynthetic phase (G_1) in dividing fibroblasts. *Anesthesiology.* 45:413-420, 1976.

Taves, D.R., Fry, B.W., Freeman, R.B., et al. Toxicity following methoxyflurane anesthesia. II. Fluoride concentrations in nephrotoxicity. *JAMA.* 214:91-95, 1970.

Taylor, G.J. Psychological factors in cancer. *Can Psychiatr Assoc J.* 19:421-422, 1974.

Tinker, J.H., Gandolfi, A.J., and Van Dyke, R.A. Elevation of plasma bromide levels in patients following halothane anesthesia: Time correlation with total halothane dosage. *Anesthesiology.* 44:194-196, 1976.

Topham, J.C., and Longshaw, S. Studies with halothane. I. The distribution and excretion of halothane metabolites in animals. *Anesthesiology.* 37:311–323, 1972.

Uehleke, H., Hellmer, K.A., and Tabarelli-Poplawski, S. Metabolic activation of halothane and its covalent binding to liver indoplasmic proteins in vitro. *Naunyn Schmiedebergs Arch Pharmacol.* 279:39–52, 1973.

Ullrich, V., and Schnabel, K.H. Formation of binding of carbanions by cytochrome P-450 of liver microsomes. *Drug Metab Dispos.* 1:176–182, 1973.

U.S. Food and Drug Administration. Guidelines for Reproduction Studies for Safety Evaluation of Drugs for Human Use, 1966, pp. 1–5.

Van Duuren, B.L., Katz, C., Goldschmidt, B.M., et al. Carcinogenicity of halo-ethers. II. Structure-activity relationships of analogs of bis-(chloro-methyl)ether. *J Natl Cancer Inst.* 48:1431–1436, 1972.

Van Dyke, R.A., and Wood, C.L. Binding of radioactivity from 14C-labeled halothane in isolated perfused rat livers. *Anesthesiology.* 38:328–332, 1973.

Van Dyke, R.A., and Gandolfi, A.J. Studies on irreversible binding of radioactivity from (^{14}C) halothane to rat hepatic microsomal lipids and proteins. *Drug Metab Dispos.* 2:469–476, 1974.

Weiman, C.G. A study of occupational stress and the incidence of disease/risk. *JOM.* 19:119–122, 1977.

Widger, L.S., Gandolfi, A.J., and Van Dyke, R.S. Hypoxia and halothane metabolism in vivo: Release of inorganic fluoride and halothane metabolite binding to cellular constituents. *Anesthesiology.* 44:197–201, 1976.

Williamson, B., Parks, N., and Samsen, L. Relative hazards to radiation workers in various classes of diagnostic x-ray procedures with special reference to ward and theatre radiography. *Aust Radiol.* 16:198–210, 1972.

Wood, M., O'Malley, K., and Stevenson, I.H. Drug metabolizing ability in operating theatre personnel. *Br J Anaesth.* 46:726–729, 1974.

6 Methods of Control

Charles E. Whitcher

Possible causal associations of health hazards in the operating room with chronic occupational exposure to trace concentrations of inhalational anesthetics has led to development of control measures which effectively reduce such exposure. Concerns related to occupational anesthetic exposure have received considerable attention only in recent years; however, the fact that that control measures were first described at least 60 years ago (Kelling, 1918) indicates the venerability of this subject. Historical aspects of waste anesthetic gases and their control are presented in Chapter 1. The present chapter is addressed to the anesthetist, dentist, and veterinarian who make use of inhalational anesthetics. It discusses sources of anesthetic gases in the operating room air and their distribution and offers a comprehensive panel of control measures. These control measures include use of low-leakage anesthetic techniques and equipment, waste gas scavenging, and air monitoring. They are safe for the patient and capable of holding occupational exposure to approximately 25 to 50 ppm nitrous oxide, with other anesthetics maintained in reduced proportionate concentrations. Such levels are reasonable to maintain and are consistent with proposed government standards (NIOSH Criteria for a Recommended Standard, 1977).

SOURCES OF ANESTHETIC EXPOSURE

Anesthetic gases are nearly always detectable in all anesthetizing locations even when no anesthetic administration is in progress. Reported concentrations during and following the administration of anesthesia were discussed earlier (Chapter 2). Sources of anesthetic gas leakage relate to the anesthetic equipment, techniques used by the anesthetist, and the patients themselves. The most obvious equipment leakages occur from the unscavenged adjustable relief valve of the carbon dioxide absorber and the unscavenged overflow valve of the mechanical ventilator. When scavenging is practiced, other leaks, such as that from the high-pressure nitrous oxide system, quickly become noticeable. This system begins at the pipeline source in the operating room and extends through the anesthesia machine as far as the flowmeters. Unfortunately, leakage from high-pressure sources is often occult, yet may produce nitrous oxide concentrations in excess of 200 ppm.

Equipment leakage is almost invariably present in low-pressure components of the anesthesia machine beginning at the flowmeters and extending through the carbon dioxide absorber, breathing tubing, breathing bag, and Y-piece connector. Such components are especially prone to leakage due to the numerous seals and joints necessary to permit disassembly for cleaning and replacement of soda lime. Anesthetic gases are soluble in both rubber and plastic which thereby provide an additional small leak source. It is unfortunate that upon usual preanesthetic examination, the low-pressure system may prove safe for the conduct of anesthesia, and yet emit high concentrations of anesthetic gases into the room air.

Leakage may occur from many other mechanical sources, including T-tubes, nonrebreathing valves, defective breathing bags, poorly designed scavenging equipment, etc. Leakage from an oxygenator used for cardiopulmonary bypass may also provide a significant source of pollution. In addition, leakage often occurs as a result of the anesthetist's techniques of administration. In many cases, this represents a lack of awareness or personal concern for occupational anesthetic exposure. This situation is unnecessary since simplified, yet safe, techniques of anesthetic administration which minimize release of anesthetic gases are readily available. Finally, the patient himself provides another anesthetic leak source since as soon as he is disconnected from the breathing system, his exhaled air inevitably disperses anesthetic gases into the operating room.

Nitrous oxide may be present in the operating room or dental operatory air during anesthetic administration in concentrations ranging from a minimum of 1 ppm to more than 1000 ppm, and halothane or other halogenated agents in concentrations from less than 0.01 to more than 20 ppm. In the operating room, an effective control program can hold average nitrous oxide concentrations to less than 5 ppm and other potent inhalation agents in proportion to those concentrations delivered to the patient. In the dental operatory, reasonably achievable concentrations may be somewhat greater. The proposed standard (NIOSH Criteria for a Recommended Standard, 1977) allows less than 25 ppm nitrous oxide in the operating room, but permits up to 50 ppm in the dental operatory.

Dental offices and veterinary clinics offer an unusual challenge in terms of finding and controlling various and unlikely sources of gas leakage. Gases may enter the anesthetizing area from remote sources in the building, such as the basement, or from outside locations where the air is heavily polluted by improperly vented suction equipment. High concentrations of gases may also occur in nonanesthetizing areas, such as the waiting room, as a result of direct mixing of gases from the adjacent anesthetizing area or carried there from remote areas by the air conditioning system.

Anesthetic exposure occurs not only in all anesthetizing locations but also in postanesthesia recovery areas. Inhaled concentrations, averaged over time, are usually lower than those in the operating room, but peak amounts inhaled by personnel directly exposed to the patient's exhaled breath can be very high, in excess of 1000 ppm. Unfortunately, highest exhaled concentrations occur upon the patient's arrival in the recovery area at a time when maximum patient care is needed.

ROLE OF AIR CONDITIONING SYSTEMS IN THE DISTRIBUTION OF ANESTHETIC GASES

Air conditioning of the surgical or dental operating room is a significant factor in occupational exposure to anesthetics. It causes widespread distribution of gases which escape into the room air; at the same time, it continuously dilutes and slowly clears gases which escape into the room. With qualifications, the air conditioning system can provide a disposal site for waste anesthetic gases.

120

Air conditioning systems fall into two main categories—recirculating and nonrecirculating (Figure 6-1). Nonrecirculating systems, also termed one-pass systems, take in fresh air from the outside and circulate cool, filtered air through the room. Whatever volumes of fresh air are introduced into the room are ultimately exhausted to the outside. Volumes are usually expressed in fresh air exchanges per hour, with a minimum of 20 such exchanges specified in most hospital building codes. Waste anesthetic gases can be efficiently disposed of via this nonrecirculating system. Gases are collected from the anesthetic breathing system through gas-tight connections, carried in appropriate transfer tubing, and deposited into the exhaust stream at the exhaust grille or farther downstream in the exhaust duct.

Recirculating air conditioning systems return part of the exhaust air back into the air intake and recirculate the mixture through the room. Thus, only a fraction of the exhaust air is disposed of to the outside. To maintain minimal levels of anesthetic exposure, air which is to be recirculated must not contain anesthetic gases; therefore, recirculating systems should not be used for waste anesthetic gas disposal. The exception is an arrangement which transfers gases into the duct at a safe distance downstream from the point of recirculation. A limitation of such a site is that positive pressure is apt to be excessive, interfering with overflow from the breathing system. At present, nonrecirculating systems are most widely used in hospitals, but

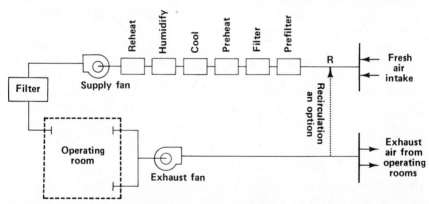

Figure 6-1 Nonrecirculating and recirculating air conditioning systems. The nonrecirculating system takes in fresh outside air, circulates it through the operating room, and then vents all of it outside. The recirculating system returns part of the exhaust air to the air intake. (From C.E. Whitcher, monitoring occupational exposure to the inhalation anesthetics. In *Monitoring in Anesthesia,* Edited by L.J. Saidman, and N.T. Smith, New York: John Wiley and Sons, 1978. Reprinted by permission of the publisher.)

availability of high-efficiency particulate air filters and the urgent necessity to conserve energy are fostering an increasing use of recirculation air conditioning. As a possible alternative, heat exchange systems can sometimes improve economy (Piziali et al., 1976).

Air conditioning systems may be further classified in terms of turbulent or laminar flow. Turbulent flow systems are the most widely used. They have relatively small inlet and exhaust grilles and high flowrates of gases. In contrast, laminar flow systems use a large air inlet, often 90% or more of an entire wall or ceiling. Large volumes of air are moved typically at a velocity of approximately 90 ft/min. Laminar flow systems recirculate the air, but because of the requirement for fresh makeup air, it has been estimated that waste anesthetic gas concentrations in the room air might be no more than 32% higher than in a standard turbulent flow nonrecirculating system (Whitcher et al., 1975). Most studies of anesthetic gas distribution have been conducted in turbulent flow systems.

Air conditioning systems effectively mix and dilute all anesthetic gas which escapes into the room. Mixing and dilution also occur in the non-air conditioned room as a result of personnel movements. Contrary to popular conception, the heavier anesthetic agents such as halothane, enflurane, and methoxyflurane do not settle to the floor, but remain mixed with the lighter gas, nitrous oxide. If mixing is complete, air samples obtained anywhere in the room contain similar concentrations of anesthetic gases. This homogeneity has been demonstrated under specific experimental and clinical conditions (Piziali et al., 1976).

Assuming uniform mixing, concentrations of gases achieved in the room air are highly predictable, as follows:

$$C = \frac{60 \times L \times 10^6}{n(L-r)V}$$

where

L = rate at which nonrecirculated anesthetic gases are introduced in liters per minute,

n = number of room air changes per hour,

r = fraction of air changes recirculated,

V = volume of room in liters.

Thus, a 3-L/min leak rate of nitrous oxide, in an operating room 20 ft square by 10 ft high provided with 10 air exchanges per hour, creates at equilibrium a room concentration of nitrous oxide of approximately 159 ppm. A leak rate of 100 ml/min yields an equilibrium concentration of 5.3 ppm nitrous oxide. Doubling the fresh-air dilution rate halves the concentration, etc.

Anesthetic gas mixing, however, may be uneven, with localized areas of concentrations above or below the average for the room. Such "hot spots" and "cold spots" impose important variables in occupational exposure. These loci of both high and low concentrations of gases present in the room air either remain in one place or move about the room, influenced by changing air distribution patterns, personnel movements, and flow obstructions such as furniture and drapes. One should be cautious in assuming a close relationship between average gas concentration in a room and that concentration inhaled by personnel. For example, the anesthetist's nose may be a short distance downstream from a very small leak source from which he or she could inhale very high concentrations of anesthetic gas. Even a minute leak in the breathing system is likely to contain at least 500,000 ppm nitrous oxide close to its source.

PATIENT SAFETY

Safety of the patient must be the prime consideration whenever anesthesia is administered. Programs directed to patient safety and programs to control occupational exposure are complementary. Preventive maintenance of equipment and leak testing procedures make for safe anesthesia. While scavenging primarily provides protection to operating room personnel, patient safety is also favored with the anesthetist unobtunded by waste anesthetic gas exposure. An air monitoring program insures that *all* control measures are effective.

Specific hazards, however, are imposed by the scavenging equipment itself and must be prevented. Misconnection of components used for scavenging the breathing system are prevented by use of non-interchangeable tubing. High pressure within the scavenging system and its reflection to the breathing system are prevented by use of collapse-resistant disposal tubing and pressure relief devices. The distal end of the disposal line must be protected from freezing and strong winds. Reexposure to the disposed gases is prevented by locating the disposal line exhaust away from personnel areas and air intakes. The explosion hazards associated with improper disposal of flammable agents are prevented by use of proper scavenging equipment designed for such agents. These hazards are addressed by the Z-79 Committee standards presently under consideration (Lecky, 1978).

CONTROL MEASURES

The objectives of the program to be proposed are to control occupational anesthetic exposure and maintain lowest reasonably achievable gas levels in the room air safely and with minimal modification of usual and customary anesthetic techniques. Costs should be modest. The program consists of six measures: (1) use of anesthetic equipment designed to be gas-tight, (2) low-leakage preventive maintenance of anesthetic equipment by qualified technicians, (3) leak testing procedures conducted regularly by in-house personnel, (4) use of low-leakage anesthetic techniques by the anesthetist, (5) efficient scavenging of waste anesthetic gases, and (6) a coordinated air monitoring program.

Low-Leakage Equipment

New anesthetic equipment should be designed by the manufacturer not only for the safe administration of anesthesia but also for gas-tight function. For example, the earlier adjustable relief valves for scavenging attachments were designed in an era preceding present standards and were far from gas-tight. Ventilators experienced a similar history with inefficient add-on scavenging attachments, until they were totally redesigned or provided with efficient gas-tight attachments. Even at the date of the present writing, scavenging equipment for the dentist is being introduced which has not received adequate clinical testing and does not scavenge efficiently. While improvements in leak tightness may add slightly to the cost of manufacture, this increase is proportionately insignificant in terms of original equipment costs.

Low-Leakage Preventive Maintenance

Preventive maintenance of anesthesia machines and ventilators performed at quarterly intervals by the manufacturer's service representative or other qualified personnel has always been good practice. Present considerations for occupational exposure require that leakage be brought to a minimum, in both the high-pressure and low-pressure components.

Particularly at the beginning of a preventive maintenance program, the high-pressure components are likely to have multiple leaks which can be difficult to locate and must be corrected. A portable nitrous oxide analyzer is useful, if not indispensable. Leakage should be reduced until the average room concentrations of nitrous oxide is 2 ppm or less. Methods of control are detailed later in the sections on leak testing and air monitoring.

The low-pressure components of gas machines, especially the carbon dioxide absorber, are vulnerable to leakage. Following quarterly

124

preventive maintenance, the measured low-pressure leak rates should be less than 50 ml/min at 30 cm water pressure.

Leak Testing Procedures

All anesthetic equipment requires frequent and regular leak testing procedures, which can be performed by trained in-house personnel. The equipment to be tested includes the anesthesia machines, ventilators, accessories associated with the breathing system, and scavenging apparatus. Concern for patient safety as well as occupational anesthetic exposure, requires leak testing of low-pressure components of the anesthesia machine prior to the induction of each anesthetic.

Potential leak sites in the absorber system are numerous and especially apt to appear following changes of soda lime. Check valves located in the low-pressure circuit may mask grossly defective anesthetic equipment (Dorsch and Dorsch, 1975). The commonly used leak test, which consists of occluding the Y-piece followed by compression of the filled breathing bag, is inadequate, and gross leakage is easily missed. Check valves are sometimes employed to prevent reverse flow into the vaporizer and may also be present in other gas circuits. It is essential to determine their presence, because even a quantitative leak test may overlook gross leakage caused by absence of a vaporizer filler cap or a broken flowmeter tube. Unless check valves are definitely known to be absent, their presence should be assumed and leak tests conducted accordingly.

The high-pressure system, as well as various low-pressure components, can also be tested by means of a bubble test. In this test, pressurization is followed by application of a soap solution or submersion in water (Figure 6-2). The test is rapid and effective in confirming suspected leak sites. The air monitoring method is a more comprehensive test because the entire system, both high- and low-pressure components, is tested as a unit, with less risk of overlooking occult sources. A rapid mobile nitrous oxide analyzer operating on battery power is ideal for this purpose.

Basic Low-Pressure Leak Test for Anesthesia Machines The following low-pressure leak test is recommended for machines without check valves and should precede induction of each anesthetic (Figure 6-3).

1. Close adjustable pressure relief valve.
2. Set oxygen flowmeter at 100 ml/min.
3. Open vaporizer control valve to ON position.
4. Occlude Y-piece.

5. Pressurize breathing system to 30 cm water using the oxygen flush valve. Attained pressure is observed on the absorber pressure gauge.

6. Make certain that pressure holds or increases over a 10-sec period.

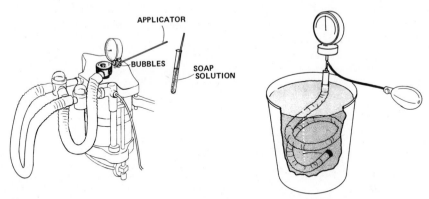

Figure 6-2 Pressurization technique for leak testing. Leakage is indicated by pressure loss and localized by gas bubbling. (From C.E. Whitcher, *Refresher Courses in Anesthesiology,* Vol. VI, Philadelphia: J.B. Lippincott, 1978. Reprinted by permission of the publisher.)

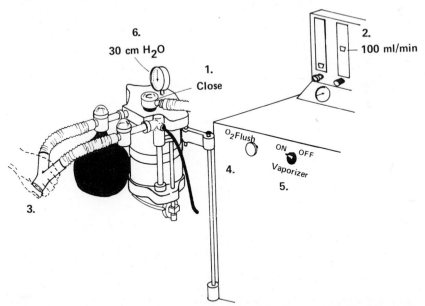

Figure 6-3 Leak tests for low-pressure components of anesthesia machines. See text.

If pressure falls, the oxygen flowmeter may be adjusted to equilibrate with and quantify leak rate. If leakage is limited to the range of 100 to 1000 ml/min, the machine may be considered acceptable for use in completing the day's schedule. Leakage exceeding 1 L/min should be repaired promptly.

Caution: A few dental machines may be damaged by pressurization. The manufacturer should be consulted to determine safe testing procedures.

Supplemental Low-Pressure Leak Test for Machines with Check Valves Perform steps 1 through 6 which precede, and maintain oxygen flow necessary to sustain pressure at 30 cm water. The machine should leak less than 1000 ml/min.

1. Momentarily, turn on, then off, each flowmeter in turn.
2. Observe a sustained increase in pressure with each on-off cycle. If pressure rise fails to occur, repair machine before use.

Leak Test for Disposal Tubing and Adjustable Relief Valve (See Figure 6-4)

1. Occlude Y-piece.
2. Open adjustable relief valve (ARV).
3. Pressurize tubing to 10 torr using oxygen flowmeter on gas machine.
4. Close adjustable relief valve.
5. Remove breathing bag from machine.
6. Observe that pressure holds for at least 10 sec.

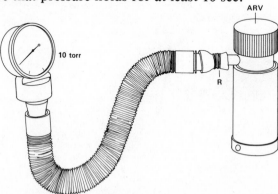

Figure 6-4 Leak test for disposal tubing and adjustable relief valve. See text. The rubber band at the pressure relief valve (R) effectively seals the temporary connection.

If pressure is slowly lost, the machine might reasonably be used, but leakage should be corrected at the end of the day's work. This test should be conducted at least once every three months.

Leak Test for High-Pressure Nitrous-Oxide Systems   The following leak test should be planned for a time when anesthetics have not been given for at least one hour. Gas machines must have had high-pressure hoses attached for a minimum of one hour. Early-morning testing is often convenient.

1. Warm up and zero the nitrous oxide analyzer (use of the nitrous oxide analyzer is discussed in the section on air monitoring).
2. Move analyzer through each room to be tested. If nitrous oxide concentration is less than 2 ppm, move to the next room. If higher concentrations are found, the sampling probe of the analyzer may be used to search for the precise source of leakage.

Repair of high-pressure leaks, of less than 2 to 5 ppm nitrous oxide may be deferred until the next scheduled preventive maintenance. Significantly higher leaks should be repaired promptly. This test should be conducted at least once every three months.

Leak Localization and Repair   If a leak is suspected, its presence should be confirmed and the exact source determined by the tests described. It should be noted that leak detection conducted with the sampling probe of the gas analyzer is a highly effective method, but may on occasion result in confusion since gas streams escaping from a leak site tend to travel and be reflected from solid obstructions and air currents.

Most leak repairs are best performed by the qualified service technician. However, the anesthetist or anesthesia technician should carry out simple maintenance measures such as determining that all gaskets are present and properly seated, making sure that tapered fittings are undamaged, and checking threaded fittings and absorber clamps for tightness. A gas-tight seal between disparate sizes of plastic and rubber tubing over metal is temporarily achievable by winding with multiple turns of tightly stretched rubber bands (Figure 6-4).

Low-Leakage Anesthetic Technique

Quality care is facilitated when the anesthetist devotes full attention to the care of the patient without unnecessary distraction. All scavenging equipment should be attached prior to the induction of anesthesia. If all attachments are completed before induction of anesthesia, the scavenging equipment should require no further attention.

The choice of anesthetic techniques should depend primarily on patient need rather than on consideration of occupational exposure. However, different anesthetic techniques are often equally advantageous. Under this circumstance, the occupational exposure factor should be carefully considered. Since the facemask is a notorious leaksource unless carefully applied, the endotracheal technique offers special advantage. When appropriate, anesthetic induction might be conducted with oxygen plus intravenous agents; inhalation agents are not started until tracheal intubation has been accomplished. The anesthetist should avoid unnecessary gas leakage, knowing that regardless of his or her personal willingness to accept the risk, other personnel who must also work in the operating room should not be exposed unnecessarily.

Specific methods for reducing occupational exposure which have proven useful in our personal practice include the following.

Before Induction of Anesthesia

1. All scavenging equipment should be attached. In many operating suites, this may be accomplished by the circulating nurse or anesthesia technician.
2. The anesthesia equipment is tested for leakage of low-pressure components using the methods described previously.
3. Vaporizers are carefully filled to minimize spillage of liquid anesthetics.
4. Nitrous oxide flowmeters are not turned on during checkout of the gas machine. Nitrous oxide is not life supporting, and failure during anesthesia is rare. The exception would be nitrous oxide circuits protected with check valves, which must be tested.
5. Gas mixtures are not sniffed to verify identity. In case of doubt, vaporizers are drained and refilled.
6. Function of breathing valves and other components can be checked by compressing the rebreathing bag prefilled with oxygen. The anesthetist should not check the anesthesia machine by breathing through the absorber system.

Induction of Anesthesia

1. Induction is accomplished with a carefully fitted face mask

which is gas-tight (gravitation techniques and loosely filled face masks result in gross leakage and may unnecessarily prolong anesthetic induction).

2. Flowmeters for anesthetic gases are turned on only after the face mask has been applied.

3. In adults, when tracheal intubation is planned, induction is usually performed with oxygen and nonvolatile anesthetic agents. Inhalation anesthetics are introduced after endotracheal intubation.

Maintenance of Anesthesia

1. Disconnection of the patient from the breathing system for tracheal intubation or suctioning is preceded by having an assistant occlude the open end of the breathing system (Figure 6-5).

2. Nonessential disconnection of the breathing system during surgery is avoided. This includes taping the endotracheal tube, and positioning the patient and the operating table.

3. The breathing bag is emptied via the scavenging system, not into room air.

4. During nitrous oxide analgesia in the dentist's chair, nonessential conversation with the patient is avoided. Exhaled nitrous oxide coming from the patient's mouth is difficult to scavenge (see section on scavenging nasal mask).

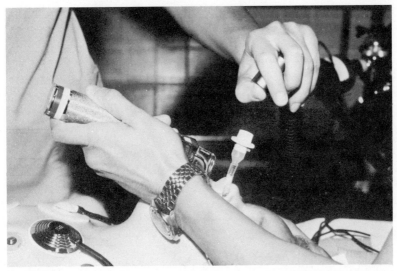

Figure 6-5 Occlusion of breathing system during tracheal intubation. The circulating nurse occludes T-piece, reducing pollution.

Recovery from Anesthesia   At the end of surgery and prior to removal of the mask or endotracheal tube, high flowrates of oxygen or compressed air are supplied to the patient to wash out the maximum amount of anesthetic agent into the scavenging system.

In the postanesthesia recovery area, the nurse must give prime consideration to patient care; when circumstances permit, the nurse might avoid the patient's exhaled gases by simple maneuvers such as moving a few inches towards the head of the bed. Occupational exposure is maximal upon the patient's arrival, but decreases rapidly.

All Phases of Anesthesia and Recovery   When conveniently available, an infrared nitrous oxide gas analyzer provides instant feedback of those techniques which cause leakage. Routine use of this monitor during each anesthetic administration is highly informative.

Waste Anesthetic Gas Scavenging

Scavenging includes collection of waste gases at the anesthetic breathing system and their disposal to the outside.

Collection of Waste Gases at the Anesthetic Breathing System Fortunately, excellent equipment is commercially available to collect waste gases from most types of anesthetic circuits. A complete scavenging unit for carbon dioxide absorber, and ventilator is shown in Figure 6-6. Since the anesthetist often switches between hand breathing and automatic ventilation, it is useful to provide a Y-piece to receive the waste gases simultaneously from the ventilator and the absorber. This arrangement permits all connections to be made before induction of anesthesia and reduces the possibility of room air pollution

Although the scavenging attachment for the Bennett ventilator is designed solely for gas disposal into the central vacuum system, this device is easily modified for other disposal methods by closing off the suction nipple. The modified Mapleson D (Bain) breathing system is easily scavenged with the Boehringer attachment.[1]

Pediatric breathing systems are also efficiently scavenged. A nonrebreathing valve with scavenging attachment is available,[2] and gas-tight devices for use with the Jackson-Rees breathing system have been developed. The arrangement shown in Figure 6-7 with the Piziali plastic wafer inserted in the bag tail is remarkably effective in protecting against accidental occlusion of the outflow tract due to twisting of the bag tail. For intermittent positive pressure breathing, the bag tail is

---

[1]Boehringer Laboratories, Inc., Wynnewood, Pennsylvania.
[2]Dupaco, Inc., San Marcos, California.

compressed with the fingers (Whitcher, 1974). The wafer must be inserted well into its lumen. Another useful method for the Jackson-Rees system is to insert a short length of semirigid plastic tubing through the bag tail and into the lumen. Positive pressure is secured by briefly occluding the intraluminal open end of the tubing via finger pressure applied through the bag wall.[3]

[3]Personal communication, J.T. Weng, New Orleans, Louisiana.

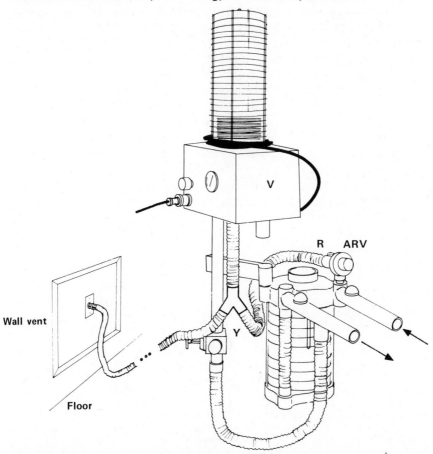

Figure 6-6 Components of a useful scavenging system. Waste gases from the adjustable relief valve (ARV) of the absorber and ventilator (V) combine at Y to enter the disposal tubing and exhaust to the outlet grille of the air conditioning system. The pressure relief valve (R) attached to the adjustable relief valve protects the patient from possible occlusion in the disposal line. (From C.E. Whitcher, *Refresher Courses in Anesthesiology,* Vol. VI Philadelphia: J.B. Lippincott, 1978. Reprinted by permission of the publisher.)

132

A gas-light attachment can be purchased[4] for the Jackson-Rees system consisting of a variable orifice rotary valve which controls outflow from the bag tail. Outflow occlusion due to twisting of the bag tail is prevented by shortening the tail and making certain that the metal tubing is inserted well into the lumen of the bag. A potential hazard in the use of this equipment is that improper control of the rotary valve may result in occlusion of the outflow and reflect excessive back pressure to the patient.

Scavenging attachments for use with pump oxygenators in cardiopulmonary bypass surgery have been described (Muravchick, 1977), but the restricted use of inhalation anesthetics for cardiac anesthesia has limited their application.

A challenging gas scavenging problem is presented for dentists who employ nitrous oxide. Dentists necessarily work very close to the patient's face, where exhaled nitrous oxide concentrations may exceed 500,000 ppm. These dentists often prefer loose application of the nasal mask, and, by intent, room air is inhaled with the nitrous oxide. Without gas scavenging, marked leakage occurs at the edges of the mask and from the valve or opening for pressure relief which is often present. Contrary to what might be expected, leakage does not necessarily occur from the patient's mouth, since the dental patient is usually carried in a light plane of analgesia with pharyngeal reflexes

---

[4]Dupaco, Inc., San Marcos, California.

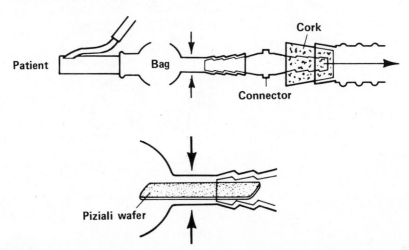

Figure 6-7 Scavenging system for the T-tube, wafer method. The wafer prevents outflow occlusion due to twisting of the bag tail. (From *Handbook of Hospital Facilities for the Anesthesiologist,* Edited by J.T. Martin, Park Ridge, Illinois: American Society of Anesthesiologists, 1974).

preserved, and the oropharynx physiologically sealed. However, gross leakage is inevitable during mouth breathing and conversation.

An effective nasal mask[5] for gas scavenging, which is essentially a mask within a mask with suction between the two mask layers, has been developed (Whitcher et al., 1977) (Figure 6-8). Leakage does not occur from this mask even when the gases are flowing and the mask is not applied to the patient. Preliminary studies of inhaled and exhaled nitrous oxide and carbon dioxide concentrations indicate effective delivery of the analgesic mixture and efficient removal of the carbon dioxide.[6] This mask must be used only with waste gas disposal by a central vacuum system.

Unfortunately, a number of inefficient dental scavenging devices have appeared on the market. The responsible manufacturer must furnish evidence of scavenging efficiency, including air monitoring studies conducted during clinical use of the equipment with nitrous oxide sampling within the dentist's breathing zone.

[5]Summit Services, Campbell, California.
[6]Unpublished studies, C.E. Whitcher, Stanford, California.

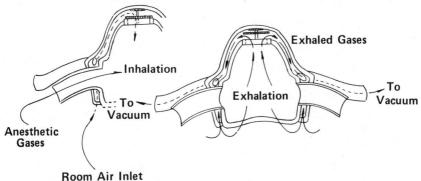

Figure 6-8 Scavenging nasal mask — The inner mask is contained within the slightly larger outer mask. The vacuum in space between the masks scavenges anesthetic gases. During normal breathing, positive pressure in reservoir bag (not shown) insures preferential inhalation of gases from anesthesia machine. During forced inhalation (negative pressure > -2 cm H_2O), machine gases are inhaled from space between masks via loosely fitted valve guide (arrow, upper left) and relief openings (not shown) located in front of outer mask. During exhalation, valve is open, and vacuum scavenges exhaled gases from the patient as well as gases leaking around the mask. (From G. Brown, Summit Services, Inc., Campbell, California. Reprinted by permission of the manufacturer.)

Waste Gas Disposal   Ideal methods for disposal of waste anesthetic gases emphasize patient safety. There must be no possibility that high pressures in the breathing system, either positive or negative, be reflected to the patient. In addition, all anesthetics, including the flammable agents, should be handled safely. The system should be inexpensive, make use of existing lines, and require no dedicated machinery. Acceptable disposal routes include the exhaust of the air conditioning system, a direct line to the outside, and the central vacuum system.

With nonrecirculating air conditioning, the exhaust grille located in the operating room provides a usable disposal site (Figure 6-6). Effluent from the breathing system is conducted through large-bore (19-mm) tubing and deposited at the grille. The sweeping effect of the airflow efficiently removes the anesthetic gases, and flammable agents are safely handled.

The air conditioning exhaust is generally considered useful for waste gas disposal only with nonrecirculating air conditioning systems. However if the system recirculates, waste gases may be disposed of beyond the point of recirculation (Figure 6-1). Unfortunately, negative pressure at this site is often excessive, greater than 10 cm H_2O, precluding its use.

Risk of accidental occlusion of the disposal line has precipitated proposed standard use of a positive pressure relief valve (Lecky, 1978). It is desirable to mount this valve close to, or directly attach it to, the adjustable relief valve of the absorber (Figure 6-6). If remote mounting is preferred, collapse-resistant transfer tubing should connect the adjustable relief valve to the positive pressure relief valve. Opening pressure of the valve shown in Figure 6-6 is 15 cm water. This appears to be the minimum pressure which easily prevents gas leakage. Lower relief pressures may be required by the proposed new standards (Lecky, 1978). *Caution:* Long lengths of tubing may be hazardous and should be kept off the floor.

An alternative method for waste gas disposal employs a direct line from the operating room to a safe outside disposal site, away from personnel areas, windows, and air intakes. As mentioned previously, a positive pressure relief valve may be required. Plastic pipe with a 1 ½-in. internal diameter has been employed in long lengths, 150 ft or more, without objectionable back pressure. Reverse flow is prevented by the normal, slightly positive pressure of the operating rooms. Flow between rooms caused by slight pressure differentials is prevented by providing each room with its own disposal line. An acceptable variation makes use of an exhaust fan which permits waste gases from more than one room to be collected into a single stack and vented to a safe disposal site. Such a system has the disadvantages of requiring machinery and pressure balancing, and must be carefully designed. The termination of these disposal lines must be protected against weather conditions (e.g., freezing) (Hägerdal, 1978) which might obstruct gas flow. Unless special provisions for dilution of flammable mixtures are provided, the method is not safe for the disposal of flammable agents.

Another variation of the direct-line disposal method provides room air dilution within the operating room (Figure 6-9). Instead of a direct connection to the disposal system, the waste gases are brought into an open receiver; a fan insures a brisk flow of room air—approximately 50 f³/min—which is evacuated along with the anesthetic gases[7]. The high flowrate insures dilution of flammable agents.

A third variation of the direct-line method makes use of a flame arrester[7] (Figure 6-10). This device is installed in the disposal line in

[7]Personal communication, K.F. Wiley, Akron, Ohio.

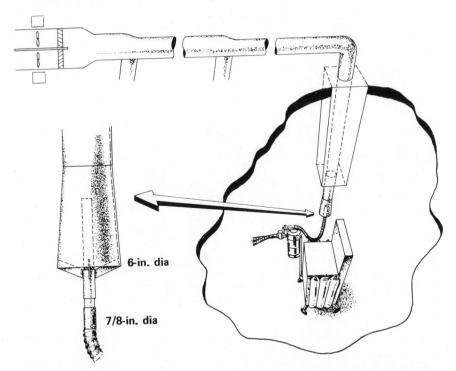

6-in. dia

7/8-in. dia

Figure 6-9 Room air dilution method for disposal of flammable and nonflammable agents. The gas mixture from the breathing circuit enters a 6-in. receiver for capture and dilution. The fan at the end of the ductwork aspirates room air and anesthetic. (From K.F. Wiley, Architect, Akron, Ohio. Reprinted by permission of Kenneth F. Wiley, AIA).

136

order to protect against fire and explosion. The flame arrester[8] is essentially a heat sink which prevents flammable mixtures from reaching ignition temperature (Glassman, 1977). Spacing between discs is critical and is set in a range of 0.16 to 0.17 mm, which appears to be the quenching distance for stoichiometric mixtures of cyclopropane in oxygen.[9] This method for fire and explosion prevention may prove useful in selected applications, although further development will be required.

In addition, the central vacuum system may be employed for disposal of anesthetic agents. To protect the safety of the patient, a positive pressure relief must be provided, and an unregulated line vacuum must not be allowed to reach the breathing system. This requires pressure balancing or interfacing. The interface (R) shown[10] (Figure 6-11) has a capacity of approximately 2L. Anesthetic gases are deposited at the bottom of the reservoir, where they are removed by suction. Efficient removal is assured when scavenging

---

[8]Protectoseal Co., Chicago, Illinois.
[9]Unpublished studies, C.E. Whitcher and A.K. Ream, Stanford, California.
[10]Boehringer Laboratories, Inc., Wynnewood, Pennsylvania.

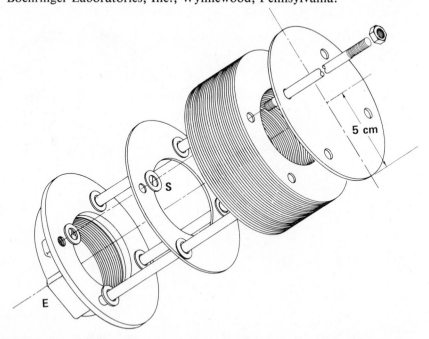

Figure 6-10 Flame arrester proposed for the disposal of flammable agents. Waste gases enter at (E) and exit between discs (S) spaced below the quenching distance.

flow exceeds fresh anesthetic gas flow, thus causing room air to enter the relief openings. Ideal application of this device includes a reservoir bag to monitor scavenging and to absorb surges in flow such as that which occurs when the breathing bag is emptied. Suction flow is monitored by a flowmeter. This device is simple, safe, and inexpensive. A limitation is that it can be used only with suction disposal, which requires machinery, electric power, and maintenance.

Compact valvular pressure relief devices have been marketed; such devices have often been unsatisfactory. Unless materials are carefully selected, valve leaflets become brittle, fit poorly, and are prone to leakage and sticking. The operating room air normally contains suprisingly large quantities of lint which can destroy valvular competence. Frequent maintenance is a necessity.

When the central vacuum system is employed, separate suction outlets for scavenging, for removal of secretions and for surgical use might be provided. However, providing 3 outlets is expensive and probably unnecessary when the complete system shown in Figure 6-11 is used. The control valve permits emergency diversion of all suction for removal of secretions. Maximum convenience is achieved by attaching all suction equipment to the gas machine, including the pressure relief system, scavenging suction flowmeter, selector valve,

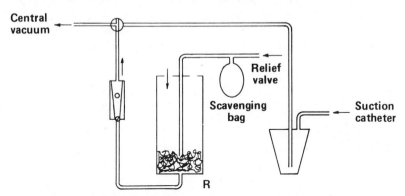

Figure 6-11 Waste gas disposal by suction. Waste gases from the breathing circuit enter the disposal system from the adjustable relief valve; surges are taken up by the scavenging reservoir bag. Gases enter the pressure relief device (R), where flow velocity is reduced by a copper-wool diffuser. Anesthetic flowmeters are set to deliver at least twice the fresh gas flowrate. This assures a continuous flow of room air through relief openings (R) (inverted arrow) and an absence of leakage. Large bore of relief openings assures pressure relief. The control valve downstream from the flowmeter diverts all suction for emergency removal of secretions. (From C.E. Whitcher, *Refresher Courses in Anesthesiology,* Vol. VI, Phildelphia: J.B. Lippincott, 1978. Reprinted by permission of the publisher and the author.

138

and patient suction bottle. All controls should be within easy reach of the anesthetist. The vacuum pump should be vented to a safe disposal site, outside the building and away from air intakes and personnel areas.

The ejector flowmeter disposal device (Figure 6-12) is widely used in Europe (Jorgensen, 1974). Compressed air or another driving gas is used in an injector configuration. The system operates economically, is safe for use with flammable anesthetics, and is independent of the air conditioning system.

Instructions provided with most scavenging equipment designed for use with the central vacuum system are labeled "Not for use with flammable agents." National Fire Protection Association Code 56A carries a similar prohibition. However, with a properly vented vacuum pump of the water-sealed type, the hazard associated with the disposal of flammable agents is acceptable.

Air Monitoring Program

All control measures discussed thus far cannot insure acceptable low anesthetic gas concentrations in the operating room air. Potential leak sources are numerous, including wall connectors, anesthesia machines, breathing circuits, and disposal systems. Leakage at these sites may be inaccessible and difficult to locate. *Final assurance of low trace gas concentrations is realized only through the use of an air monitoring program.*

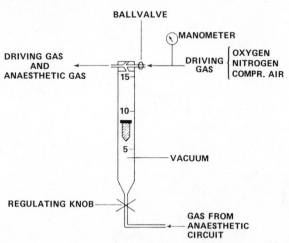

Figure 6-12 Ejector flowmeter method of waste gas disposal. Waste gases are entrained in a compressed air stream. (From Jorgensen, *Acta Anaesthesiol Scand.* 18:29–33, 1974. Reprinted by permission of Munksgaard International Publisher, and of the author.

Gases to be Monitored   Theoretically, an ideal air monitoring program would monitor all gases used. Analyzers are available which continuously scan the infrared spectrum and are programmable to distinguish individual inhalation anesthetics;[11] however, it is simpler to monitor a single gas. Nitrous oxide is a logical choice for monitoring, considering its ease of measurement and almost universal use.

The Tracer Concept   The tracer concept suggests that, under specified conditions, relative proportions of anesthetic agents are similar in the breathing circuit and in the room air. When the anesthetic equipment is relatively gas-tight, most gases in the room air originate from the breathing system due to residual leakage within the components or as a result of the anesthetist's technique. Gases entering the room air are diluted, but their relative concentrations remain the same. Knowing the concentration of any one inhalation anesthetic in room air, the concentrations of any other anesthetic in use can be readily calculated. For example, anesthetic mixtures achieved with 3 L/min nitrous oxide and 2 L of oxygen with halothane 0.05 L/min contains nitrous oxide and halothane in a ratio of 60:1. If the measured room concentration of nitrous oxide is 60 ppm, the room concentration of halothane is approximately 1 ppm.

The tracer concept holds best under conditions of steady-state anesthesia and tightly controlled equipment leakage. The concept does not apply while the vaporizer is being filled, when the high-pressure nitrous oxide hose is disconnected, or during the induction and recovery phases of anesthesia. However, these phenomena are transient. Figure 6-13 shows simultaneous measurements of nitrous oxide and halothane under clinical conditions. Parallelism of concentrations is apparent.

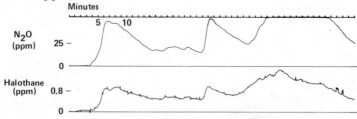

Figure 6-13   Simultaneously recorded N_2O and halothane. Differences between channels are related to instrumental differences and sensitivity settings. Gases are sampled at the air conditioning exhaust grille. (Figures 6-13 through 6-18 from C.E. Whitcher and R.L. Piziali, *Anesth Analg. (Cleve),* 56:778–785, 1977. Reprinted by permission of the International Anesthesia Research Society.)

---

[11]Foxboro/Wilks, East Norwalk, Connecticut.

Methods of Gas Analysis (The Infrared Gas Analyzer)   Several methods of gas analysis should be considered. Air samples may be sent to a commercial laboratory which supplies necessary sampling equipment and directly reports concentrations of both nitrous oxide and potent agents.[12,13] A serious disadvantage of this approach is inevitable delay in the reporting of results. The precise circumstances of sampling are likely to be forgotten, and the effect of corrective measures cannot be assessed immediately. Moreover, analysis of a large number of samples is expensive. An alternative method is in-house gas anlaysis. The available infrared nitrous oxide analyzers are satisfactory and readily obtainable.[14–18]

Operation of the infrared analyzer depends upon a unique spectrum of absorption peaks for each gas. A strong absorption peak for nitrous oxide is present at 4.45 micrometers (μ). Halogenated anesthetics have absorption peaks at 8.9 μ and 12.4 μ, but not at 4.5 μ; carbon dioxide may interfere with nitrous oxide analysis because of its near-coincident peaks at 4.3 μ. As a result, precautions must be taken to avoid the high concentration of carbon dioxide present in expired air. Infrared analyzers are also sensitive to water vapor likewise present in high concentrations.

A diagram of a typical infrared analyzer (Figure 6-14) shows a pump which continuously perfuses the sample cell with nitrous oxide and air. The infrared source generates a light beam which is filtered to pass only those infrared components specific for nitrous oxide. This beam is transmitted through the windows of the sample cell and is sensed by the detector. The higher the concentration of nitrous oxide in the cell, the greater the absorption of infrared light and the lower the energy level at the detector. The resultant signal is processed and displayed as ppm of nitrous oxide.

Operation of the nitrous oxide analyzer with battery power presents significant advantages in permitting rapid survey of all rooms in the suite. Time is also saved in eliminating the need for attaching the power cord and warming up the instrument each time it is moved from room to room.

All analyzers must be calibrated. Instrumental zero is established by perfusing the sample cell with a noninfrared absorbing gas such as

[12]Air Test Labs., Inc., Rochester, New York.
[13]Boehringer Laboratories, Inc., Wynnewood, Pennsylvania.
[14]Air Products and Chemicals, Inc., Allentown, Pennsylvania.
[15]Cavitron KDC Corp., Anaheim, California.
[16]Foxboro/Wilks, East Norwalk, Connecticut.
[17]Ohio Medical Products, Madison, Wisconsin.
[18]Sensors, Inc., Ann Arbor, Michigan.

compressed air, oxygen, or clean air. (The air conditioning inlet provides a convenient source for the latter, but only with nonrecirculating systems). Sensitivity is calibrated with a standard gas mixture purchased in cylinders, or custom mixed (Figure 6-15). This method is essentially a closed system which includes the sample cell of the analyzer. Injection of carefully measured quantities of pure gas, such as nitrous oxide, permits preparation of standard gas concentrations. For routine use, a single-point calibration is sufficient.

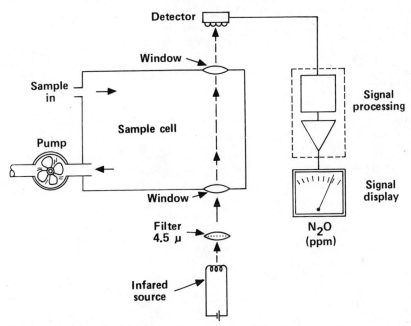

Figure 6-14 Infrared analyzer for N_2O. The sample for analysis enters the sample cell and varies the amount of infrared light transmitted. The resultant signal is displayed in ppm N_2O.

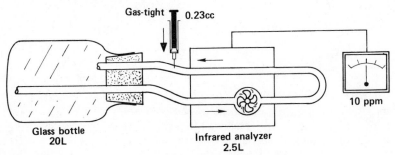

Figure 6-15 Method for calibrating gas analyzers.

Infrared analyzers with variable or interchangeable filters[19] are capable of measuring all infrared absorbing gases, including the halogenated anesthetics. Unfortunately, analysis of these agents is fraught with technical difficulties. The simpler infrared analyzers do not distinguish among the several potent halogenated agents. Results are also subject to interfering substances often present in the operating room, including isopropyl alcohol, formalin, ammonia, freons, and organic iodides used in skin disinfection. These technical difficulties favor an air monitoring program based on the tracer concept and the analysis of nitrous oxide alone.

Air Sampling Techniques   The sampling technique used is critical in obtaining samples representative of actual gas concentrations inhaled by personnel. An important consideration is that anesthetic gas leakage is apt to be intermittent (Figure 6-16). Nitrous oxide concentrations shown vary from 5 to 97 ppm. Leakage variations make for difficulty in obtaining single grab samples representative of actual inhaled concentrations. Better representation of average inhaled concentration is obtained by collecting the sample in a gas-tight bag or charcoal tube filled at a constant rate over time. Analysis of the contents provides a time-weighted value. Despite their precision, such methods are cumbersome for routine monitoring.

---

[19]Foxboro/Wilks, East Norwalk, Connecticut.

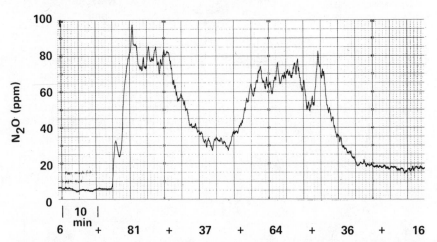

Figure 6-16   Typical N_2O leakage patterns during anesthesia. The waveform is determined by the output of the N_2O analyzer during anesthesia provided by the face mask. The sampling site is the exhaust grille of the air conditioning system. The average of perpendiculars gives the time-weighted average for the case—N_2O = 40 ppm.

A viable method of time weighting is to average the results of a series of grab samples. Many such samples, obtained with the infrared analyzer at varying hours each day, achieve the necessary randomization. Alternatively, the output of the nitrous oxide analyzer can be integrated by taking the average of perpendiculars drawn at equal intervals (Figure 6-16). Time-weighted values obtained by this method are similar to the bag sample method in the tracing shown. Integration may also be accomplished electronically.

Air samples obtained within the breathing zone of personnel are most likely to represent the gas concentrations actually inhaled, and are usually preferred. The breathing zone is defined as an area in a frontal plane within 6 to 10 in. of the nose or at the midpoint of the clavicle. Breathing zone sampling is to be distinguished from general area sampling. Area sampling is justifiable only when it has been clearly demonstrated through multiple gas measurements that gases are evenly distributed in the room. When leakage is under effective control, gas concentrations may be similar throughout the operating room. If so, area sampling is appropriate.

Uses of the Infrared Analyzer   The infrared analyzer for nitrous oxide has multiple uses in the operating room. It can assess occupational exposure, enhance patient safety, instruct operating room personnel as to sources of leakage, and indicate successful repair. Leakage in the entire high-pressure nitrous oxide system is determined by survey of the operating suite. Specific methods are listed in the previous section on leak testing.

Results of a high-pressure leak survey in one hospital are shown in Figure 6-17. Operating rooms in the suite are noted on the horizontal axis, and nitrous oxide concentrations are shown on the vertical axis. It is apparent that significant leakage is present in room 1. Only a few days earlier, this room evidenced a nitrous oxide concentration of only 1 ppm. Leakage was localized to a crack in the nitrous oxide line at the rear of the anesthesia machine. This machine was otherwise serviceable for clinical anesthesia. The leak was not audible, and in the absence of a high-pressure survey, it would have gone undetected for a long time.

Nitrous oxide concentrations determined during clinical anesthesia measure total leakage, including leaks related to the techniques of the anesthetist, as well as high- and low-pressure components of the anesthesia machine and the ventilator. For this survey, the analyzer is best operated on battery power and moved into each operating room in sequence. If the breathing-zone nitrous oxide concentration is low, i.e., less than 25 ppm, the result is recorded and the analyzer moved to the next room. If a high value is obtained, the analyzer may be employed as a leak detector (Figure 6-18). As an example of the analyzer's contribution to patient safety, the earliest warning of patient disconnection in the breathing system has been observed repeatedly as a rise in the room concentration of nitrous oxide. As an example of the analyzer's contribution to anesthesia training, the student can be instructed objectively in the techniques for gas-tight application of the face mask.

The frequency with which air monitoring is conducted is an important consideration. Proposed NIOSH standards suggest a three-month interval to coincide with the proposed requirement for quarterly preventive maintenance. More frequent monitoring may be necessary at the inception of the anesthetic waste gas control program. At this time, it is especially useful to have available an infrared analyzer. Larger hospitals might justify cost of their own instruments; smaller suites might obtain an instrument by leasing. As alternatives, commercial agencies that perform preventive maintenance might also do the air monitoring, or samples could be sent to an outside laboratory.

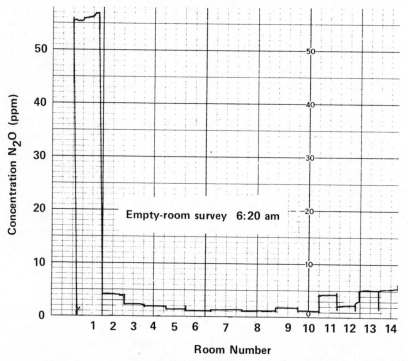

Figure 6-17 Room survey for high-pressure N_2O leakage. "Clean" operating rooms not in use have less than 1 to 2 ppm N_2O.

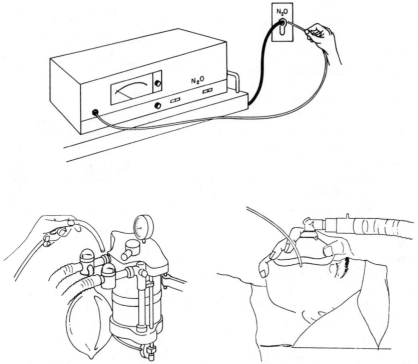

Figure 6-18 Use of nitrous oxide analyzer as a leak detector. The sampling probe of the analyzer is directed toward suspected leak sites.

Control Measures Not Recommended

Control measures not recommended include increasing the normal fresh-air exchange rate of the air conditioning system, venting gases to the floor level, and using charcoal absorbers.

Both closed-circuit and low-flow anesthetic techniques have been proposed as acceptable alternatives to scavenging. Inherent advantages include reduced atmospheric[20] pollution and lower costs (Virtue, 1978). With closed techniques, anesthetic gases are not released into the room air, and scavenging is theoretically superfluous. However, few anesthetists confine themselves to the totally closed system, and in the absence of scavenging, anesthetic gases may be released during the induction and recovery phases of anesthesia, etc. Low-flow techniques without scavenging obviously result in the continuous release

---

[20]The term *atmospheric* in relation to pollution properly refers to the outside air.

of small volumes of anesthetic gases into the room air. If anesthetic exposure is to be held to a minimum, it is apparent that even with the closed-system and low-flow techniques, scavenging should be a routine practice.

Discussions concerning the relationships of anesthetic gas flowrates to scavenging often overlook important phases of the control program. Exposure is minimized only when all control measures are practiced, including the use of well-maintained, low-leakage equipment and techniques supported by air monitoring and scavenging.

Increasing the fresh-air dilution rate of the air conditioning system decreases anesthetic exposure but is not cost-effective. Venting the waste gases to the floor level is also ineffective because the air conditioning flow quickly distributes even the heaviest agents throughout the room. Charcoal cannisters effectively adsorb the potent anesthetics, but nitrous oxide adsorption is negligible.

Costs to Control Occupational Exposure

Necessary costs to initiate and maintain a control program must take into account the potential health benefits. As discussed in earlier chapters, the hazards are significant, and adequate control measures may well reduce their risk, although this remains to be proven.

Initial low-leakage preventive maintenance of an anesthesia machine may require two to three hours of technician time; subsequent maintenance should be completed within an hour. Many leak testing procedures may be performed by in-house personnel and are fully justifiable on the basis of patient safety.

An adjustable scavenging pressure relief valve in 1979 costs approximately $120; a positive pressure relief valve[21] sells for as low as $30; a scavenging nasal mask costs approximately $150 plus installation; a ventilator with scavenging attachment could be bought for approximately $1000; and older ventilators can be converted for scavenging at modest cost. The cost of a disposal system is highly variable. If the air conditioning exhaust grille is used, the cost is determined by the length of collapse-resistant tubing. If concealed lines are installed in conjunction with remodeling, costs attributable to the scavenging system are also minimal. If a dedicated central vacuum system has to be specifically installed, high costs are incurred. Gas samples analyzed by an outside laboratory cost $20 to $40 per sample. An infrared nitrous oxide analyzer costs approximately $3500.[22]

---

[21]G. Dundas Co., Black Diamond, Washington.
[22]All dollar amounts in this paragraph are approximate figures for 1979.

Procedures in Organizing a Control Program

A program might be first initiated by measuring uncontrolled gas concentrations prevailing in the suite. An active program would then develop with purchase and installation of new leakproof equipment as replacements are needed. A low leakage preventive maintenance program and training of personnel in leak testing procedures and in low-leakage anesthetic techniques could follow. Evaluation of the effectiveness of these efforts would be achieved through use of a nitrous oxide gas analyzer. It is important that personnel exposed to anesthetics in all anesthetizing locations and in postanesthesia areas be informed of the possible health risks involved. This is a proposed requirement in the NIOSH criteria for a recommended standard and would seem both morally and legally justified.

CONCLUSIONS

Anesthetic exposure can be held to a minimum with reasonable ease and relatively minor costs. It would seem only reasonable to protect exposed personnel since significant potential health hazards may exist in all anesthetizing areas.

REFERENCES

Dorsch, J.A., and Dorsch, S.E. *Understanding Anesthesia Equipment: Construction, Care, and Complications.* Baltimore, Maryland: Williams and Wilkins Co., 1975

Glassman, I. *Combustion.* New York: Academic Press, 1977.

Hägerdal, M., and Lecky, J.H. Anesthetic death of an experimental animal related to a scavenging system malfunction. *Anesthesiology.* 47:522–523, 1978.

Jorgensen, S. The injector flowmeter and its clinical application. *Acta Anesthesiol Scand.* 18:29–33, 1974.

Kelling, G. Uber die beseitigung der narkosedampfe aus dem operationssaale. *Zentralbl Chir.* 45:602–606, 1918.

Lecky, J.H. Chairman, American National Standards Institute, Committee Z-79. *SC-4 Anesthesia Gas Scavenging Devices and Disposal Systems.* Draft, March 1978.

Muravchick, S. Scavenging enflurane from extracorporeal pump oxygenators. *Anesthesiology.* 47:468–471, 1977.

National Institute for Occupational Safety and Health. *Criteria for a recommended standard: Occupational exposure to waste*

148

anesthetic gases and vapors. DHEW Publication No. (NIOSH) 77-140. Cincinnati, Ohio, 1977.

Piziali, R.L., Whitcher, C., Sher, R., et al. Distribution of waste anesthetic gases in the operating room air. *Anesthesiology.* 45:487–494, 1976.

Virtue, R.W. Anesthetic gas flows, costs, and pollution: Some personal reflections. *Anesth Rev.* 5:14–16, 1978.

Whitcher, C., Cohen, E., and Trudell, J. Chronic exposure to anesthetic gases in the operating room. *Anesthesiology* 35:348–353, 1971.

Whitcher, C. Control of waste anesthetic gases. Edited by J.P. Martin. In *Handbook of Hospital Facilities for the Anesthesiologist.* The Committee on Hospital Planning and Construction, American Society of Anesthesiologists, Park Ridge, 1974.

Whitcher, C., Piziali, R., Sher, R., et al. Development and evaluation of methods for the elimination of waste anesthetic gases and vapors in hospitals. GPO stock no. 1733-0071. Superintendent of Documents, Government Printing Office, 1975.

Whitcher, C.E., Zimmerman, D.C., Tonn, E.M., et al. Control of occupational exposure to nitrous oxide in the dental operatory. *J Am Dent Assoc.* 95:763–776, 1977

7 Role of Federal Government

Charles L. Geraci, Jr.

Historical perspectives surrounding occupational exposure to inhalation anesthetic agents have been discussed in Chapter 1. It is sufficient to state here that the problem has been a topic of scientific interest and debate for many years, beginning with the report by Hirsch and Kappus (1929) and continuing to the present. The following discussion outlines activities of the two federal government agencies concerned with this issue—the National Institue for Occupational Safety and Health (NIOSH) and the Occupational Safety and Health Administration (OSHA). Although the mission and duties of these agencies differ, both organizations are concerned with health and welfare of the United States workforce.

The Occupational Safety and Health Act of 1970, Public Law 91-596, was passed by Congress to assure, insofar as possible, every working man and woman in the nation safe and healthful working conditions and to preserve our human resources. The Act created NIOSH as an agency of the Department of Health, Education and

Welfare and charged it with specific aspects of public health authority and responsibility. Major among NIOSH mandates are: (1) to conduct and fund research and studies for determining the effect of chronic or low-level exposure to industrial materials, processes, and stresses for their potential to cause illness, disease, or loss of fundamental capacity; (2) development of criteria for recommended standards which describe safe exposure levels for varying periods of employment, including, but not limited to, that exposure level at which no employees will suffer impaired health or functional capacities or diminished life expectancy as a result of their work experience.

While conducting its research, NIOSH may make workplace investigations, interview employers and employees, as well as measure and report employee exposure to potentially hazardous materials. As a result of research conducted or sponsored by NIOSH, substances may be determined to be potentially toxic at the concentrations in which they are found or used in a place of employment. If such substances are not covered by an occupational health standard, or if an existing health standard is found not to be sufficiently protective, NIOSH is charged to submit this determination, together with all pertinent criteria, to OSHA. Created by the Occupational Safety and Health Act as an agency of the Department of Labor, OSHA has among its major responsibilities (1) to encourage employers and employees to reduce hazards in the workplace and implement new or improve existing safety and health programs; (2) to establish separate, but dependent responsibilities and rights for employers and employees for the achievement of better safety and health conditions; (3) to establish reporting and record-keeping procedures to monitor job-related injuries and illnesses; (4) to develop mandatory job safety and health standards and enforce them effectively. The duties and responsibilities of both NIOSH and OSHA relevant to the issue of occupational exposure to waste inhalation anesthetics will be elaborated in the following paragraphs.

NIOSH RESEARCH

NIOSH first became involved in the issue of chronic exposure to inhalation anesthetics in December 1971, when members of the Institute met with the National Academy of Sciences National Research Council Ad Hoc Committee on Adverse Reactions to Anesthetic Agents. The purpose of the meeting was to review preliminary health surveys conducted in Russia, Denmark, and the United States which suggested that women working in operating rooms and chronically exposed to trace concentrations of anesthetic gases and vapors were experiencing an increased rate of spontaneous abortion. These early studies generated significant interest in the potential health hazards and in the development of means of controlling exposure to waste anesthetic gases and vapors. The waste anesthetics resulted from the inadvertent release of gases and vapors of volatile liquid anesthetics into the work area during administration of inhalation anesthesia. The potential adverse health effects associated with chronic exposure to waste anesthetics led NIOSH to sponsor a workshop in Salt Lake City in June 1972. The intent of this workshop was to have members of the professional anesthesia societies, health and hospital associations, and concerned scientists evaluate all potential health hazards associated with chronic exposure to waste anesthetics.

One of the most significant results of the workshop was initiation of a program of scientific investigation to evaluate these potential occupational problems associated with chronic exposure to waste anesthetics. NIOSH provided contractual funding to the American Society of Anesthesiologists (ASA) for the conduct of this formidable investigation. Subsequently the ASA established its Ad Hoc Committee on the Effect of Trace Anesthetics on the Health of Operating Room Personnel and a national health survey of operating room personnel and dentists was undertaken. The intent of the survey was to document the health histories of those individuals indentified as experiencing chronic exposure to waste anesthetics. The investigation surveyed approximately 57,000 members of professional health-care associations who experienced chronic exposure to the operating room and to waste anesthetics, using approximately 24,000 members of two nonexposed associations as control groups (Cohen et al., 1974). Major findings indicated an increased incidence of embryotoxicity, teratogenesis, and female carcinogenesis among operating room personnel. The results of this large study confirmed and added to the findings of the growing list of smaller studies that suggested an increased occurrence of miscarriage and birth defects among operating room-exposed personnel.

NIOSH contracts were later awarded to Northwestern University to assess potential effects of trace concentrations of anesthetics on behavioral performance in operating room personnel (Bruce and Bach, 1976). Evaluated in these studies were the effects of nitrous oxide and halothane on vigilance, visual perception, memory, and audiovisual coordination and reaction time. Exposure concentrations studied were those in the operating room both with and without effective control measures for waste anesthetic gases. Although these studies monitored extremely subtle health effects, the investigators were able to document a measurable performance decrement among exposed volunteers at exposure concentrations encountered in a hospital operating room or dental office.

A questionnaire survey of approximately 1200 hospitals was subsequently conducted by NIOSH in order to obtain representative information concerning anesthetic practices. Major areas included identification of the anesthetics and their extent of use, methods of administering anesthesia, and methods currently used to reduce exposure of operating room personnel to waste anesthetics. The information gathered in this survey was used to assist in formulation of appropriate work practices and engineering control procedures developed under another phase of the total effort and is presented in the NIOSH criteria document.

Additional NIOSH contracts were awarded to Stanford University to conduct pilot research programs in the development and evaluation of methods for eliminating waste anesthetic exposures (Whitcher et al., 1975). Not only were engineering control methods developed and evaluated, but a program of anesthetist work practices was formulated which could help reduce levels of waste anesthetics. Development of an air monitoring program to test the effectiveness of mechanical control procedures and anesthetist work practices was also undertaken. Work was also initiated to develop means for monitoring and controlling exposure to nitrous oxide in dental offices (Whitcher et al., 1977).

A NIOSH contract was also awarded to the Hazelton Laboratories to conduct inhalation studies in the experimental animal with both nitrous oxide and halothane. The primary goal of this study was to evaluate reproductive, teratogenic, and mutagenic effects, as well as investigate the reported increased incidence of malignancies following chronic anesthetic exposure. The study was carried out in several phases (Coate, Kapp, and Lewis, 1979). The first phase assessed the effect in rats of chronic exposure to two inhaled concentrations of nitrous oxide plus halothane on the incidence of reticuloendothelial malignancies. Histopathologic evaluation of selected tissues was conducted following different periods of exposure. The data indicated that long-term exposure of rats to mixtures of nitrous oxide plus halothane did not result in an increase in the incidence of neoplasia nor a specific increase in the incidence of reticuloendothelial tumors.

The second phase of the Hazelton study investigated effects of long-term exposure to nitrous oxide plus halothane on reproductive performance of female rats and development of their offspring. Mated female rats when exposed to combinations of halothane and nitrous oxide demonstrated reduced ovulation and implantation efficiency and slightly retarded development of their fetuses. The reported increased incidence of miscarriage seen in human health surveys was not strictly paralleled in the rats. The major significance of this aspect of the study was to indicate that chronic exposure to halothane and nitrous oxide, at likely encountered concentrations, may exert toxic effects on reproduction, and is therefore of concern.

The final phase of the Hazelton study involved cytogenetic evaluation of bone marrow and spermatogonial cells in male rats following long-term exposure to nitrous oxide plus halothane. Based on the data obtained, it was concluded that chronic exposure to halothane plus nitrous oxide at trace concentrations usually encountered in their use as inhalation anesthetics can cause chromosomal damage to bone marrow cells in the rat. The cytogenetic evaluation of spermatogonial cells in male rats also revealed chromosomal damage following this chronic exposure.

NIOSH CRITERIA DOCUMENT

The preceding paragraphs describe the means by which NIOSH began the task of meeting its legislative mandate to conduct and fund research investigations concerned with potential health hazards in the workplace. NIOSH is also required by Section 20 of the Occupational Safety and Health Act to develop and transmit to OSHA criteria which describe exposure levels to toxic materials that are safe so that the Department of Labor is, in turn, able to meet its responsibility for the formulation of safety and health standards.

One of the ways in which recommendations are transmitted to OSHA is in the form of a NIOSH criteria document. These documents, which are published by NIOSH, are prepared from an evaluation of published or publicly available medical, biologic, engineering, and chemical information. The evidence is critically reviewed to determine which hazardous effects are relevant in developing criteria for the proposed standards. A criteria document receives thorough review by personnel of NIOSH and other Federal agencies, by occupational health consultants experienced with the subject of the document, and by professional societies whose membership includes professional personnel experienced in occupational health or familiar with specific matters presented in the document. Following final review by senior NIOSH personnel and approval by the director, the criteria document is transmitted to the Department of Labor, OSHA.

As a result of the information gathered, NIOSH identified several major areas of potential concern regarding chronic exposure to waste anesthetics. Of prime concern were the reports of adverse effects on reproduction among exposed operating room personnel. Increased spontaneous abortion rates and increased incidences of congenital abnormalities among children of exposed nurses and anesthetists were the most frequently reported adverse health effect. Also reported and reviewed were studies indicating an increased incidence of liver and kidney disease among exposed personnel, especially female workers. Reports of an increased rate of cancer among exposed female personnel also generated a level of concern. In addition to the hospital-based information reviewed by NIOSH, limited data were also gathered among general dentists and dental oral surgeons. For those dentists identified as being exposed to inhalation anesthetics in the dental operatory, there was an increased incidence of spontaneous abortion among their wives, and an increased incidence of liver disease among the dentists themselves.

Having identified several major potential health hazards which could result from chronic exposure to waste anesthetics, NIOSH undertook the task of identifying the population at risk. The most logical place to find exposed workers is, of course, the hospital operating room. The average surgical procedure requiring inhalation anesthesia frequently involves four to seven persons. Included in this exposed group are the surgeon, anesthetist, operating room nurse, circulating nurse, and operating room technician. NIOSH prepared estimates of the number of patients anesthetized each year in all hospitals in order to quantify the potential for exposure. These estimates indicated that approximately 20 million patients are anesthetized annually in the nearly 25,000 hospital operating rooms in the United States. An average of 800 anesthetics is conducted in each operating room per year. Considering the average composition of the surgical team, it is likely that hospital operating rooms may be responsible for 3200 to 5600 anesthetic exposures per year.

Another method used to estimate the number of potentially exposed personnel combined the population figures of the various professional groups involved with those activities directly related to occupational exposure. For hospital operating room exposure to waste anesthetic gases, the following data are useful: American Society of Anesthesiologists, 15,000 members; American Association of Nurse Anesthetists, 17,500 members; Association of Operating Room Nurses, 25,000 members; and the Association of Operating Room Technicians, 13,000 members. The 70,500 potentially exposed workers listed here do not include surgeons, students, volunteers, or recovery room, labor, or delivery room personnel.

Hospital personnel are not the only individuals exposed to waste anesthetics. Many general dentists and oral surgeons use inhalation anesthetics to produce anesthesia or analgesic sedation. An estimate made by the American Dental Association and the American Society of Oral Surgeons suggests that approximately 35,000 to 40,000 dentists use nitrous oxide on a routine basis. A smaller proportion regularly use nitrous oxide plus halothane. This estimate does not include dental assistants who are also exposed. The American Dental Assistants Association has a membership of approximately 25,000, and it is estimated that in this group alone, 10,000 to 15,000 assistants may be potentially exposed. The nonaffiliated dental assistant group is even larger (probably five times this number), bringing the total number of exposed dental assistants to between 50,000 and 75,000 individuals.

Personnel in veterinary medicine are also exposed to waste anesthetics. Although this group has received less attention, similarities in the practice of anesthesia in human and animal hospitals create essentially the same exposure for veterinarians and their assistants as for hospital operating room personnel. Estimating exposures in veterinary medical practice is difficult, but the American Veterinary Medical Association suggests that in its membership of 28,000 individuals, there are as many as 50,000 veterinarians and their assistants potentially exposed. Based on all of the estimates presented it is possible that as many as 200,000 individuals are potentially exposed in the U.S. alone.

Once an estimate of the extent of exposure had been obtained, attempts were made to quantify the exposure. A number of reports have appeared in the literature indicating the concentrations of anesthetics found in an operating room during the conduct of anesthesia (Chapter 2). NIOSH was not only interested in documenting exposure concentrations, but was also concerned with developing a reliable means of air monitoring. From the available data, it appeared that the average hospital operating room concentration of halothane ranged from 1 to 10 ppm and that of nitrous oxide from 400 to 3000 ppm. Data obtained from dental offices indicated much higher anesthetic concentrations than in hospitals, especially for nitrous oxide. Concentrations of nitrous oxide in dental offices thus ranged from 500 ppm to as much as 7000 ppm and were as high as 200 ppm in the waiting room and office areas. Air monitoring would appear to be the only means of determining the effectiveness of any control measure that might be taken to reduce waste anesthetic exposure. The development of an effective, reliable monitoring program is thus of great value in determining the effectiveness of control procedures and work practices.

When sufficient information had been gathered and key projects completed, development of a criteria document on waste anesthetics was initiated. As noted, NIOSH is mandated to develop criteria for use by OSHA in establishing occupational health standards. In developing the criteria document, NIOSH recognized that the adverse effects on reproduction among operating room personnel chronically exposed to waste anesthetics were of primary concern in the development of a recommended standard to control such exposures. Liver disease rates among exposed personnel and the decrement in performance following experimental exposures to anesthetics were also factors in development of the recommended standard. The question of possible carcinogenicity of certain anesthetic agents was a concern during review of the data both because of the reported increased cancer rate among exposed female personnel and because of a similarity in structure between certain of the halogenated anesthetics and known human carcinogens. However, data available from animal exposure studies were judged equivocal, and the information could serve only as a warning and as an indication for future study. The recommended standard was transmitted to the Department of Labor, OSHA, in March 1977 (Criteria for a Recommended Standard, 1977).

The criteria document contains five major aspects. These are the recommended standard itself, data on the biologic effects of exposure, data on extent and degree of exposure, information on past and current control procedures and work practices, and available methods for monitoring concentrations of waste anesthetics in the room air. A critical point emphasized in the criteria document is that none of the recommended control procedures is intended to preclude proper patient care and safety.

The recommended standard is intended to suggest allowable air concentrations in the workplace that are safe based on available health data. NIOSH, however, considered that a safe level of exposure to waste anesthetics could not be defined due to the equivocal nature of many of the animal exposure studies and certain of the human health surveys. An additional difficulty in both the animal and human health data lies in the possible combinations of halogenated anesthetics, nitrous oxide, or mixtures of the anesthetics. When the halogenated anesthetics are used alone, the recommendation is that occupational exposures be controlled so that no worker is exposed to concentrations greater than the minimum levels that can be determined with reasonable ease, reliability, and reproducibility. That concentration was judged to be a time-weighted average (TWA) of 2 ppm of any halogenated anesthetic agent sampled from the ambient air during the entire period of anesthetic administration using charcoal adsorption and gas chromatographic analysis. When halogenated agents are used in combination with nitrous oxide, the recommendation is that exposures be controlled to the lowest concentrations easily and feasibly attained with currently available control technology. It was determined that a TWA concentration of 25 ppm nitrous oxide during the period of administration is feasible. Controlling the mixed anesthetic agents to this level will result in a TWA of approximately 0.5 ppm for the halogenated agents. Special treatment was given to those situations where nitrous oxide is the sole agent used, i.e., primary use in dentistry.

Recommendations are also made for control procedures and work practices aimed at minimizing exposure to waste anesthetics. The prime recommendation is that anesthetic delivery systems be equipped for scavenging so that waste gases can be conducted away from the work area. Specific recommendations are also made regarding fitting of various breathing systems with adequate scavenging equipment, use of pressure balancing devices, and a means of conducting the collected waste gases to an adequate disposal site.

Anesthetist work practices recommended in the document carry the intent of reducing exposure by making key personnel in the operating room aware of means by which this can be accomplished. Recommended also are procedures for determining proper operation of scavenging equipment, leak testing of the low-pressure end of the breathing circuit, leak testing of associated equipment, as well as suggested work practices before and after delivery of the anesthetic agents. This section of the recommended standard is vital to the reduction of anesthetic exposures. Merely installing a scavenging device does not constitute an adequate control program. A regular program of testing and maintaining of the equipment is necessary, in addition to the use of the work practices aimed at minimizing exposures. Responsibility for implementing the majority of control procedures, tests, and work practices most naturally falls upon the anesthetist.

Other aspects of the recommended standard are concerned with areas of medical surveillance of exposed employees, employee information and education, and record-keeping requirements and monitoring requirements. Medical surveillance is recommended, but not manditory. Medical records that are maintained should be periodically updated. Employees are to be informed of the possible health effects of exposure to waste anesthetics as reported in the literature and are to be instructed as to the availability of this information. Record-keeping requirements state that records and results of monitoring, corrective measures taken, and medical surveillance be maintained. Based on the standard practice of record retention, where a question of potential carcinogenicity exists, a record retention period of 20 years is recommended. Air monitoring is recommended to be conducted on a quarterly basis in areas representative of employee exposure during anesthetic administration. Breathing-zone samples obtained from exposed employees are the most desirable, but are not mandatory. Specific information on control procedures and air monitoring was presented in Chapters 2 and 6. Although specific methods of sampling and analysis are detailed in the criteria document, any method demonstrating equivalent precision and accuracy is acceptable for monitoring.

OSHA STANDARDS

With transmittal of the NIOSH criteria document to the Department of Labor, the first phase of NIOSH's investigations ends and involvement by OSHA can begin. OSHA can initiate standard setting procedures in a number of ways, but relies heavily on NIOSH investigations, research, and technical support. Once OSHA has developed plans to propose, amend, or delete a standard, these intentions are published in the *Federal Register* as a "Notice of Proposed Rulemaking," or often as an "Advance Notice of Proposed Rulemaking." The notice includes terms of the new rule and provides a specific time (at least 30 days from the date of publication, occasionally 60 days or more) for the public to respond.

Interested parties who submit written arguments and pertinent evidence may request a public hearing on the proposal when none has been announced in the notice. When such a hearing is requested, OSHA must schedule and publish in advance the time and place in the *Federal Register*. Within 60 days after close of the comment period or public hearing, OSHA must publish its ruling in the *Federal Register,* along with the full and final text of any standard amended or adopted and the date the new ruling will become effective.

No decision on a permanent standard is reached without due consideration of the arguments and data received from the public in written submissions and at hearings. However, if any affected party, employer, or employee believes that a final standard or rule is too burdensome, is inadequate, or does not reflect the record in the case, an appeal may be made (within 60 days of the rule's publication) to the U.S. Circuit Court of Appeals for the circuit in which the objector lives or has his or her principal place of business. Filing an appeals petition, however, will not delay the enforcement of a standard, unless the court of appeals specifically orders it.

Current scientific information, as well as the thinking of those active in the field, indicates that there would be much discussion and argument surrounding proposed rule making by OSHA regulating exposure to waste anesthetics. Many feel that there are additional experiments and health surveys that must first be conducted before thought be given to drafting a legal standard. However, should a permanent standard be issued and new information become available relevant to the basis for the standard, there are still mechanisms for input. OSHA continually reviews and redefines its safety and health standards as industrial technology and safety and health knowledge continue to develop. Therefore, employers and employees should be aware that, just as they may petition OSHA for the development of standards, they may also petition OSHA for standard modification or revocation.

OSHA Enforcement

Assuming a permanent standard for occupational exposure to waste anesthetics is adopted, the next item of interest is the relative priority that hospitals, or any other location using inhalation anesthetics, will be given for inspection. Imminent danger situations are obviously given top priority. An imminent danger is any condition where there is reasonable certainty that there exists a danger that can be expected to cause death or serious physical harm immediately or before the danger can be eliminated through normal enforcement procedures. This may not be the case with waste anesthetics, since nearly all data indicate situations of low-level, chronic exposure. A high priority could be placed on waste anesthetic exposures if a definite correlation is demonstrated between chronic exposure and long-term health efforts. Second priority is given to investigation of catastrophes, fatalities, and accidents resulting in hospitalization of five or more employees. Third priority is given to valid employee complaints of alleged violation of standards or of unsafe or unhealthful working conditions.

The Occupational Safety and Health Act gives each employee the right to request an OSHA inspection when the employee feels he or she is in imminent danger from a hazard or when he or she feels OSHA standards are being violated. OSHA will inform the employee of any action it takes regarding the complaint and, if requested, will hold an informal review of any decision not to inspect. Voluntary compliance will undoubtedly be a major factor in this issue since many hospitals, because of various governmental affiliations, fall outside the jurisdiction of OSHA.

Responding to employee complaints will be the mechanism most likely used by OSHA in initiating waste anesthetics inspections. A hospital health inspection for waste anesthetics may consist of a team of OSHA compliance officers conducting appropriate air sampling for nitrous oxide and halogenated anesthetics as well as meeting with the hospital administration and interviewing employees. After the compliance officers report to the OSHA office, the area director determines what citations, if any, will be issued and what penalties, if any, will be proposed. Penalties associated with citations are usually monetary. When issued a citation or notice of proposed penalty, an employer may request an informal meeting with the OSHA area director. This written notification is termed a Notice of Contest. The OSHA area director then forwards the case to the independent Occupational Safety and Health Review Commission. The commission assigns the case to an administrative law judge. The judge may investigate and disallow the contest if it is found to be legally invalid, or a hearing may be scheduled to be held in a public place as close as possible to the employer's workplace. The employer and the employees have the right to participate in the hearing. The review commission does not require that they be represented by attorneys. Once the administrative law judge has ruled, any party to the case may request further review by the review commission itself. Any of the three commissioners also may, at his or her own motion, bring a case before the commission for review. If the commission issues its own ruling, that ruling may itself be appealed to the U.S. Circuit Court of Appeals for the circuit in which the case arose.

General Duty Clause

Although a waste anesthetics standard has not as yet been promulgated, it is still possible for OSHA to conduct inspections in hospitals or any facility that uses inhalation anesthetics. Section 5(a)(1) of the Occupational Safety and Health Act, known as the general duty clause, states that an employer is responsible for furnishing a place of employment free from recognized hazards. It is possible, therefore, for OSHA to respond to complaints by hospital employees about working conditions, even in operating rooms.

In one recent situation, operating room personnel in a Cincinnati hospital complained to the OSHA area director regarding adverse health effects they associated with their workplace. The operating room nurses and technicians complained of heat stress, dizziness, and fatigue. They were aware of many of the waste anesthetic gas epidemiologic studies. OSHA sent in a team of industrial hygienists who conducted a walk-through inspection and air sampling. It was noted that the operating room was equipped with scavenging for halogenated anesthetics, but not for nitrous oxide. In sampling the air of three different operating rooms, the inspectors found the highest concentrations of nitrous oxide to be 333 ppm measured during a 141-minute operation. The NIOSH criteria document recommends 25 ppm as the permissible exposure limit. The inspection resulted in two separate, but identical citations for both the hospital administration and a group of seven anesthesiologists. In issuing its citation to the anesthesiologists, the OSHA area director indicated that the anesthesiologists had definite knowledge of the hazard; the group had attended conferences on the hazards of waste anesthetic gases. The director felt that responsibility for controlling exposure was up to the group having control over the area and not solely that of the hospital administration.

Soon after the Cincinnati inspection, the OSHA regional office in Philadelphia conducted four hospital inspections which resulted in two citations, one in Bethlehem and one in Harrisburg. It is reasonable to assume that based on OSHA's willingness to respond to hospital employee complaints, such inspections will continue in the future.

ONGOING STUDIES

Much information concerning health hazards and control of waste anesthetics remains to be gathered and evaluated. NIOSH is continuing to conduct significant efforts. An ongoing activity within NIOSH that has provided valuable assistance to hospitals, dental offices, and veterinary clinics is the Health Hazard Evaluation program. Under this program, a hospital administration or group of employees can request an investigation by NIOSH to assess potential health hazards and conduct an environmental investigation. Many hospital hazards evaluations have already been conducted by the institute. The most valuable assistance so far appears to be the air sampling program conducted by NIOSH industrial hygienists, with subsequent recommendations made to hospitals regarding control procedures and establishment of an air monitoring program. NIOSH is also attempting to keep information current by publishing revisions to its earlier documents. These revisions contain the latest information pertaining to hospital control procedures as well as control procedures relevant to veterinary anesthesia practices.

In keeping with an admitted limited amount of information concerning the health experience of dentists and their assistants, and in terms of its research responsibilities, NIOSH has funded a study through its grants process to gather this information. A recent grant awarded to Stanford University is to be used to identify and conduct a health survey among dentists and chairside assistants chronically exposed to inhalation anesthetics. NIOSH also continues to provide support for investigations into the biologic effects of exposure to waste anesthetics and has recently funded two animal studies. The first study, funded at the American Dental Association Health Foundation, will attempt to further assess and characterize possible biologic effects of exposure to nitrous oxide. The second study, being conducted at Duke University, will investigate possible increases in toxicity of trace anesthetics caused by ultraviolet light. It is hoped that these studies will provide important additional information in areas remaining to be addressed in a comprehensive and critical evaluation of the issue of waste anesthetic gases.

REFERENCES

Bruce, D.L., and Bach, M.J. *Trace effects of anesthetic gases on behavioral performance of operating room personnel.* DHEW Publication No. (NIOSH) 76-169. Cincinnati, Ohio: U.S. Department of Health, Education and Welfare, National Institute for Occupational Safety and Health, 1976.

Coate, W.B., Kapp, R.W., Jr., and Lewis, T.R. Chronic low-level halothane-nitrous oxide exposure: Reproductive and cytogenetic effects in rats. *Anesthesiology* 50:310-318, 1979.

Coate, W.B., Ulland, B.M., and Lewis, T.R. Chronic low-level halothane-nitrous oxide exposure: Lack of carcinogenic effect in rats. *Anesthesiology* 50:306-309, 1979.

Cohen, E.N., Brown, B.W., Bruce, D.L., et al. Occupational disease among operating room personnel: A national study. *Anesthesiology.* 41:321-340, 1974.

Hirsch, J., and Kappus, A.L. On the quantities of anesthetic ether in the air of operating rooms. *Z Hyg.* 110:391-398, 1929.

National Institute for Occupational Safety and Health. *Criteria for a recommended standard: Occupational exposure to waste anesthetic gases and vapors.* DHEW Publication No. (NIOSH) 77-140. Cincinnati, Ohio, 1977.

Whitcher, C.E., Piziali, R., Sher, R., et al. *Development and evaluation of methods for the elimination of waste anesthetic gases and vapors in hospitals.* DHEW Publication No. (NIOSH) 75-137. Cincinnati, Ohio: U.S. Department of Health, Education and Welfare, National Institute for Occupational Safety and Health, 1975.

Whitcher, C.E., Zimmerman, D.C., Tonn, E.M., et al. *Control of occupational exposure to nitrous oxide in the dental operatory.* DHEW Publication No. (NIOSH) 77-200. Cincinnati, Ohio: U.S. Department of Health, Education and Welfare, National Institute for Occupational Safety and Health, 1977.

8 Medical–Legal Implications

Gale A. Mondry

During the last decade, there has been increasing awareness of the tremendous human and economic loss occasioned by occupational diseases. In response, legislation and legal principles have been developed to clarify the respective rights and duties of employers and employees with regard to occupational safety and health issues. Recent studies suggest that health professionals exposed repeatedly to anesthetics have an increased risk of spontaneous miscarriage, congenital deformities, liver and kidney disease, and cancer in females. This chapter will discuss the impact of recent legal developments upon institutions and individuals affected by the potential health hazards of anesthetic exposure.

OCCUPATIONAL SAFETY AND HEALTH ACT OF 1970

The most comprehensive piece of legislation pertaining to workplace hazards is the Occupational Safety and Health Act of 1970

(OSHA). The stated purpose of OSHA is ". . . to assure so far as possible every working man and woman in the nation safe and healthful working conditions and to preserve our human resources."[1] To accomplish this, the act places upon employers various responsibilities. The following section outlines the general requirements of OSHA and analyzes how these requirements may be applied to situations involving occupational exposure to waste anesthetics.

Administration and Enforcement

Under the terms of OSHA, an employer is required (1) to furnish each of its employees employment and a place of employment which are free from recognized hazards that are causing or are likely to cause death and serious physical harm to employees, and (2) to comply with occupational safety and health standards duly promulgated by the Secretary of Labor.[2]

To insure that employers fulfill their responsibilities, OSHA created a complex enforcement mechanism. The Secretary of Labor acts as both the "legislator" and "prosecutor." The Secretary of Labor legislates by promulgating OSHA standards. Currently, there are thousands of health and safety standards. In addition to promulgating specific health and safety standards, the Secretary of Labor requires each employer to adhere to a general duty of care to his or her employees, i.e., to furnish a place free from recognized hazards.

As prosecutor, the Secretary of Labor reviews whether employers are in compliance with OSHA's general duty clause and the requirements of specific OSHA standards. The Secretary is given the authority to inspect all workplaces, and employees may initiate an inspection by filing a written request with the Department of Labor. During the course of an inspection, representatives of the employer and employees are given an opportunity to accompany the inspector, in order to assist in the discovery of workplace hazards. Subsequent to the inspection, if the Secretary believes there are violations of OSHA, the Secretary will issue a citation setting forth the alleged violations and fixing a reasonable time for their elimination. In addition, the Secretary will provide notice of the proposed penalty for any OSHA

---

[1] 29 U.S.C.A. Section 651(b)(1975).
[2] OSHA also requires that employers prepare and maintain various records of occupational injuries and illnesses; however, employers that employ no more than 10 full-time or part-time employees are relieved from such record-keeping requirements.

violation. The size of the proposed penalty depends upon the severity of the violation.[3]

An employer may challenge the citation, the proposed penalty, or the abatement date by filing a notice of contest within 15 working days from receipt of the proposed assessment of penalty. An employee has the right to challenge the reasonableness of the abatement period provided by the secretary. If no challenge is filed within 15 days, the citation and assessment become a final order, not subject to review by any court or agency.

In the event of a challenge, a full hearing is held before the independent Occupational Safety and Health Review Commission (OSHRC), which consists of three individuals appointed by the President of the United States with the advice and consent of the Senate. The OSHRC, through its administrative law judges, decides whether to affirm, modify, or invalidate the Secretary of Labor's citation or proposed penalty. Thereafter, any person adversely affected by an order of the OSHRC, including the Secretary of Labor, may appeal OSHRC's decision to the appropriate federal court of appeals. OSHRC's decision will be sustained by the reviewing court if supported by substantial evidence.

Application of OSHA to Situations Involving Occupational Exposure to Anesthetics

No Specific Standard Governing Such Exposure Under OSHA, there are three kinds of specific standards that may be promulgated: interim standards, permanent standards, and temporary standards. Currently, the Secretary of Labor has not promulgated any type of health and safety standard regulating occupational exposure to anesthetic gases.

OSHA vests in the Secretary of Labor the discretion to determine whether a standard should be published and what its particular contents should be, but the Act does set forth some basic guidelines. In promulgating standards dealing with toxic materials or harmful physical agents, the standard, whenever practicable, should be expressed in terms of objective criteria and of the performance desired. The standard should prescribe the use of labels or other appropriate forms of warning to insure that employees are apprised of all hazards

---

[3]For example, nonserious violations carry penalties of up to $1000, whereas willful or repeated violations carry penalties of up to $10,000.

to which they are exposed, relevant symptoms, appropriate emergency treatment, and proper conditions and precautions of safe use or exposure. The standard should provide for control or technological procedures to be used in connection with such hazards and for monitoring or measuring employee exposure at such locations and intervals and in such manner as may be necessary for the protection of employees. In addition, where appropriate, a standard should prescribe the type and frequency of medical examinations which should be made available by the employer to employees exposed to such hazards in order to most effectively determine whether the health of such employees is adversely affected by exposure. The results of such examinations shall be furnished only to the Secretary of Labor, to the Secretary of Health, Education and Welfare, and, at the request of the employee, to the employee's physician.[4]

Within 60 days after the issuance of an OSHA standard, any person may challenge the validity of the standard in the appropriate federal court of appeals. OSHA states that the Secretary of Labor's standards shall be upheld if supported by substantial evidence in the record considered as a whole. Most courts, however, recognizing that the Secretary is often making policy determinations rather than factual conclusions, have, in fact, given more deference to the Secretary's standards than would seem to be called for with the substantial evidence test.[5]

The Secretary of Labor has not published a health and safety standard prescribing minimum exposure levels to waste anesthetics and setting forth necessary warnings, monitoring procedures, and medical examinations. However, the process for developing such a standard has been initiated. In March 1977, the National Institute for Occupational Safety and Health (NIOSH) published a recommended standard governing occupational exposure to waste anesthetic gases and vapors.[6]

NIOSH was created by OSHA under the auspices of the Department of Health, Education and Welfare. NIOSH functions include, among others, developing and establishing recommended occupational safety and health standards. Any standard recommended by NIOSH is immediately forwarded to the Secretary of Labor. Some

[4]29 U.S.C.A. Section 655(b)(1975).

[5]*Industrial Union Department, AFL-CIO* vs *Hodgson,* 499 F.2d 467 (D.C. Cir. 1974); *Synthetic Organic Chemical Manufacturers Ass'n* vs *Brennan,* 503 F.2d 1155 (3rd Cir. 1974).

[6]*Criteria for a Recommended Standard . . . Occupational Exposure to Waste Anesthetic Gases and Vapors.* National Institute for Occupational Safety and Health, DHEW (NIOSH) Publication No. 77–140, March 1977.

have argued that once the Secretary decides to issue regulations, NIOSH's criteria are binding to the extent feasible; however, courts have held that NIOSH criteria are merely advisory.[7]

Because the NIOSH document does not constitute a promulgated OSHA standard, employers are not obligated to comply with its recommendations. No standards governing exposure to waste anesthetic gases and vapors currently exist, and, therefore, an employer could not be in violation of a specific OSHA standard by exposing employees to high levels of waste anesthetics.

Ultilization of the General Duty Clause In addition to requiring compliance with specific health and safety standards, OSHA imposes upon employers the broad general duty of providing a place of employment free from recognized hazards which are causing or are likely to cause death or serious physical harm. Employers can be cited for a violation of this general duty clause of OSHA even though they have not breached any of the specific OSHA standards.

The elements which must be present to constitute a violation of the general duty clause are more complex than those involved in the violation of a specific OSHA standard. To demonstrate a breach of an OSHA standard, the Secretary of Labor must only show that a standard exists, that the employer has not complied with the standard, and that this noncompliance has a direct relationship to safety and health.[8] When relying on the general duty clause, the secretary must demonstrate that (1) employees are being exposed to a hazard, (2) the hazard is a recognized one, because either the employer had knowledge that the condition was hazardous, or else the condition was recognized as hazardous in the industry as a whole, (3) the hazard is likely to cause death or serious physical harm, with the test being one of plausible rather than probable harm, and, (4) there exist feasible methods of reducing or eliminating the recognized hazard which the employer failed to undertake.[9] Common law defenses such as assumption of risk or contributory negligence are not of use to an employer charged with an OSHA violation.[10]

In more than one case, the Secretary of Labor has taken the position that an employer that exposes its employees to high levels of waste anesthetics is in violation of OSHA's general duty clause. The case which proceeded the farthest involved the Bethesda Hospital in Cincinnati, Ohio. On August 16, 1977, after receiving a complaint from

---

[7]*Industrial Union Department* vs *Hodgson, supra,* note 5.
[8]*Lee Way Motor Freight, Inc.* vs *Secretary of Labor,* 511 F.2d 864 (10th Cir. 1975).
[9]*National Realty and Construction Co.* vs *OSHRC,* 489 F.2d 1257 (D.C. Cir. 1973).
[10]*REA Express, Inc.* vs *Brennan,* 495 F.2d 822 (2nd Cir. 1974).

operating room personnel, compliance officers from the Department of Labor's Occupational Safety and Health Administration (OSHA) conducted an inspection of the Bethesda Hospital operating rooms. It was found that no engineering controls such as exhaust ventilation or scavenging methods had been implemented for reducing the levels of nitrous oxide released during the administration of anesthetic gases. In addition, monitoring procedures had not been instituted to determine the levels of nitrous oxide or halogen gases present in the operating room during the administration of anesthetic gases. As part of its inspection, the OSHA investigators measured the exposure levels of some individuals and found them to be in excess of the levels recommended in the NIOSH criteria document.[11]

As a consequence of its investigation OSHA notified Bethesda Hospital on October 21, 1977 that it was being cited for a serious violation of the Occupational Health and Safety Act of 1970. The citation stated that because of the hospital's "failure to monitor and institute control measures the employees had been subjected to the potential hazards associated with these gases which include chronic effects such as spontaneous abortion and congenital abnormalities in their offspring; liver and kidney disease; central nervous system damage and acute effects such as headache, nausea, and fatigue." OSHA proposed a penalty of $490 for the citation and indicated that by December 21, 1977, a ventilation system should be installed in the hospital's operating rooms and regular monitoring should be implemented. On November 8, 1977, the hospital notified OSHA that it intended to contest the citation, proposed penalty, and methods and dates of abatement.

Bethesda Hospital, along with the group of anesthesiologists who practiced there, maintained that the OSHA citation was unjust. They stated that exposure to waste anesthetics could not be termed a "recognized hazard" since research on the effects of anesthetics was very recent and as yet inconclusive. In addition, they argued that there

---

[11]Specifically, the results of their tests showed that: (1) the anesthesiologist in O.R. No. 4 was exposed to a concentration of Ethrane of 2.78 ppm during a 48-L/48-min sample, and to an Ethrane concentration of 2.38 ppm during a separate 47-L/47-min sample; (2) the anesthesiologist in O.R. No. 4 was exposed to a concentration of nitrous oxide of 333.5 ppm during a 141-min sampling period; (3) the anesthesiologist in O.R. No. 3 was exposed to an Ethrane concentration of 2.78 ppm duing a 46-L/46-min sample; (4) the anesthesiologist in O.R. No. 3 was exposed to a nitrous oxide concentration of 123.8 ppm during a 51-min sampling period; and, (5) the scrub nurse in O.R. No. 3 was exposed to a concentration of Ethrane of 2.25 ppm during a 52-L/52-min sample.

were no established guidelines concerning safe and unsafe levels of waste anesthetics nor any official guidelines on the methods to use for maintaining desired levels of concentration. Further, they indicated that conditions at Bethesda Hospital were no different from those which existed at most of the surrounding Cincinnati hospitals.

It was the Department of Labor's position that exposure to anesthetics at the level found in the Bethesda Hospital operating rooms did constitute a recognized hazard. Articles on the potential health hazards of exposure to anesthetics had been published in well-known medical journals, such as the *Journal of the American Medical Association, Anesthesiology,* and *Lancet,* which were readily accessible to the medical community. Moreover, the Bethesda Hospital anesthesiologists knew of the contents of the NIOSH criteria document which included extensive information regarding the potential hazards of occupational exposure to anesthetics. Although no OSHA standard was applicable, the department maintained that the procedures at Bethesda Hospital were so inadequate—no ventilation system, no monitoring, exposure levels up to 13 times the recommended NIOSH standard—that the hospital, as well as the private-practice anesthesiology group, could be cited for an OSHA violation based upon its failure to comply with the Act's general duty clause. The argument that other hospitals had routinely failed to institute adequate control measures was said to be irrelevant.

The Bethesda Hospital case was set for a hearing before an administrative law judge of OSHRC. However, on July 27, 1978, prior to the administrative hearing, the parties reached a settlement. Under the terms of the settlement, the citation issued against the anesthesiologists was withdrawn, the hospital certified that it had installed a ventilation and monitoring system to abate the cited conditions, and the proposed penalty against the hospital was reduced to $25.

As stated before, the Bethesda Hospital case proceeded farther than any other similar citation. There are as of this date no OSHRC or court decisions dealing with the validity of an OSHA citation for failure to take adequate measures to control the exposure of employees to waste anesthetics. There are, however, court cases dealing with other types of citations under the OSHA general duty clause which suggest that a citation in the Bethesda Hospital situation may have been appropriate. In one case, a reviewing court upheld the citation under the Act's general duty clause of an employer for exposing its employees to hazardous airborne concentrations of lead. The court said that when an employer was allegedly violating a health standard that had been recognized in the industry for years, but a particular OSHA standard was not yet applicable, a citation could nonetheless be issued under the Act's general duty clause.[12] In another case, involving a general duty citation for the accumulation of titanium dust, a court rejected an employer's argument that there was no precise standard establishing what level of accumulation was likely to cause death or serious physical harm. The court stated that the "fact that no precise standard exists as to what level of accumulation is dangerous in the Section 5(a)(1) sense, far from relieving petitioner of the burden of minimizing accumulation, arguably imposes an even greater duty on petitioner, faced with the obligation of taking feasible measures to assure the safety of its employees, to err, if at all on the side of the greater, not lesser, caution."[13]

Responsible Parties OSHA places upon an employer the primary responsibility for providing a safe and healthful place of employment to its employees, and sets forth sanctions which can be imposed if this duty is not met. The Secretary of Labor has taken the position that an employer will be cited for an OSHA violation only when the employer's own employees are exposed to unsafe or unhealthful conditions. This policy raises some troublesome questions at work sites with more than one employer.

In the hospital operating room, several employers are involved. Typically, only the nurses who work in the operating room are employed by the hospital. The anesthesiologists and surgeons who practice in the operating rooms are not hospital employees. These physicians are employers themselves and have individuals working for them—e.g., nurses, secretaries, bookkeepers—but their employees perform their duties in the physician's offices and not in the hospital.

Since the hospital has employees in the operating room who are potentially exposed to the hazard of anesthetics, the hospital is an appropriate party to cite for a violation under OSHA. Some commentators have criticized the Secretary of Labor's reliance on exposure as the sole criterion for citation at multiemployer work sites and have indicated that instead, those employers who caused the hazard and/or have the ability to eliminate the hazard should be held liable under the Act.[14] A few courts have moved toward the adoption of this latter approach at least in cases concerning nonserious violations. In either event, a hospital would be subject to citation under OSHA because its employees are exposed to the potential health hazards of occupational

---

[12]*American Smelting and Refining Co.* vs *OSHRC,* 501 F.2d 504 (8th Cir. 1974).

[13]*Titanium Metals Corporation of America* vs *Usery and OSHRC,* 6 OSHC 1873 (9th Cir. 1978).

[14]B. Fellner and D. Savelson, *Occupational Safety and Health: Law and Practice,* New York: Practicing Law Institute, 1976.

exposure to anesthetics and because it has the ability to install scavenging and monitoring systems which would assist in abating the potential hazard.

The OSHA liability of the involved anesthesiologists does depend on whether or not employee exposure is the criterion for citation. In the hospital operating room setting, employees of the anesthesiologists are not being exposed to anesthetics.[15] However, anesthesiologists do bear some of the responsibility for the creation of excessive levels of waste anesthetics in the operating room and have some control over abatement of the potential hazards. This is true because the work practices of anesthesiologists can contribute to the presence of waste anesthetic gases. Specifically, the failure to properly connect and utilize scavenging equipment, the use of ill-chosen or ill-fitting endotracheal tubes, and the use of gases when the breathing system is disconnected from the patient increase the level of waste anesthetics. Furthermore, since only one group of anesthesiologists usually practices in a particular hospital, it is easier to attribute some of the responsibility to that private practice group than it would be if several different groups, each of which had different work practices, administered the hospital's anesthesia.

The Bethesda Hospital case does not clarify the issue of physician liability for an OSHA citation. The private practice anesthesiology group was cited along with Bethesda Hospital for an OSHA violation. However, as part of the settlement, the citation against the group was withdrawn, and the group was not required to pay a penalty or take any corrective action.

Review of the NIOSH Criteria for Occupational Exposure to Waste Anesthetics

In March 1977, NIOSH published its recommendations for a specific OSHA standard governing occupational exposure to waste anesthetic gases and vapors. If the Department of Labor decides to promulgate regulations on this subject, NIOSH recommendations will undoubtedly be given close consideration. The NIOSH recommendations are divided into nine sections: (1) definitions, (2) workplace air, (3) control procedures and work practices, (4) medical, (5) labeling and posting, (6) fire, explosion, and sanitation practices,

---

[15]This would not be the case if anesthetics were administered in the offices of an anesthesiologist, dentist, or veterinarian and the personnel involved in assisting in the anesthetic's administration were their employees.

(7) informing employees of hazards from anesthetic gases, (8) monitoring requirements, and (9) record-keeping requirements.[16] In many ways, these recommendations resemble already-existing OSHA standards which regulate exposure to other toxic substances such as asbestos and vinyl chloride.

The definitions section makes it clear that the NIOSH recommendations pertain to occupational exposure to anesthetics which occurs not just in hospital operating rooms but also in dental offices, veterinary medical areas, and hospital delivery, labor, and recovery rooms. This is so, despite the fact that most of the human studies conducted and reported at the time the NIOSH recommendations were published dealt with hospital operating room personnel. Nonetheless, NIOSH stated that the health effects of chronic exposure to waste anesthetic gases in other anesthetizing locations could be similar.

The NIOSH recommendations detail the maximum concentrations of anesthetics to which a worker should be exposed—no more than 2 ppm of any halogenated anesthetic agent, based on the weight of the agent collected from a 45-L air sample by charcoal absorption over a sampling period not to exceed one hour; no more than 25 ppm of nitrous oxide at time-weighted average (TWA) concentrations during the anesthetic administration period. This approach comports with the requirements of OSHA that, whenever practicable, standards dealing with toxic materials should be expressed in terms of objective criteria.

In the third section of the recommended standard, employers are required to undertake a number of actions designed to minimize exposure to waste anesthetics. For example, scavenging devices or ventilation systems are required, and various leakage tests are described for equipment used in administering anesthetics. The inclusion of a section on control procedures is also suggested by the Act itself which states that, where appropriate, standards should prescribe suitable protective equipment and control or technological procedures to be used in connection with the hazards.

The fourth section of the NIOSH recommendations concerns the delicate subject of medical surveillance of employees. The recommendations state that comprehensive preplacement medical and occupational histories should be obtained and maintained in an employee's medical record and that the information contained therein should be updated at least annually. An employee's medical records should also contain the results of recommended preplacement and annual

---

[16]*Criteria for a Recommended Standard . . . Occupational Exposure to Waste Anesthetic Gases and Vapors, supra,* note 6.

physical examinations as well as documentation of any abnormal outcomes of the pregnancies of the employee or of the spouse of the employee exposed to anesthetic gases. Employers are to maintain these medical records for the period of the employee's employment plus 20 years. Copies of an employee's medical record are to be available to the designated medical representatives of the Secretary of Health, Education and Welfare, the Secretary of Labor, the employer, and the employee or former employee.

Virtually all OSHA standards dealing with hazardous or toxic substances contain provisions on medical examinations and records. In this context, two particular issues have been debated at some length: (1) providing the results of medical examinations to the employer without the consent of the involved employee, and (2) providing copies of an employee's medical records to government agencies without the consent of the involved employee.

The case of *Industrial Union Department, AFL-CIO* vs *Hodgson, supra,* concerned a challenge to the Secretary of Labor's OSHA standard for occupational exposure to asbestos dust. Among other complaints, employees maintained that the standard which provided the employer with access to the results of employee medical examinations should be modified so that these results were available to the employer only with the consent of the employee. The Court of Appeals, noting that employees were not required to undergo medical examinations, upheld this portion of the asbestos standard because it said employers were required to take into consideration the health of their employees in making job assignments.

The NIOSH recommended standard on medical surveillance of employees occupationally exposed to anesthetics is similar to portions of the asbestos dust standards which were upheld as a legitimate exercise of the Secretary of Labor's rule-making authority. There are some differences, however. The NIOSH recommendations require that the results of employee medical examinations be available only to the "designated medical representative" of the employer. Nothing is said about the right of the medical representative to release this information to other individuals, such as an employee's supervisor who might have responsibility for job assignments. In addition, it is unclear whether the NIOSH provisions concerning the maintenance of medical and occupational histories and documentation of pregnancy outcomes are mandatory or elective. Because of the private nature of this information, it would seem best to give employees the choice of supplying the information.

Since the publication of the NIOSH criteria document, the Department of Labor has proposed a model standard for regulating exposure to toxic substances. In this proposed model standard, the section on medical surveillance provides that the employer shall make available to its employees comprehensive medical examinations, but these examinations shall not be mandatory. After conducting a medical examination, the examining physician furnishes an opinion on stated topics to the employer with a copy to the employee, but the physician's opinion should not reveal specific findings or diagnoses unrelated to occupational exposure.[17] Future regulations concerning medical surveillance of employees occupationally exposed to anesthetics may follow this format.

Another issue which has arisen in a few cases has concerned the availability of employees' medical records to representatives of a government agency such as NIOSH. In one case, *E.I. du Pont de Nemours and Company* vs *Finklea*,[18] NIOSH was conducting a research investigation at one of du Pont's plants to determine whether any substance normally found at that plant had potentially toxic effects in such concentrations as used or found. As part of its investigations, NIOSH wished to determine whether there was a high incidence of cancer among employees at the plant and, if so, whether such incidence was job related. NIOSH, therefore, issued an administrative subpoena to the manager of the du Pont plant asking him to produce the personnel and medical records of all former and current employees of the du Pont plant. Du Pont corresponded with approximately 3000 of its past and present employees, asking them to indicate whether they consented to the release of their medical records. Of the employees who responded, 1717 gave their consent to the proposed disclosure, and 631 refused. Du Pont declined to disclose to NIOSH the medical records of the 631 employees who did not consent to disclosure. This occasioned a lawsuit over the validity of the subpoena. The court upheld the NIOSH subpoena. It found that NIOSH was conducting a legitimate investigation and that the medical information sought was relevant to its inquiry. Assuming without deciding that an employee had a right to privacy in his or her medical record, the court held that this right would not be invaded impermissibly by such disclosure. NIOSH had assured the court that the information would be treated confidentially and when not in active use, would be kept in a locked vault. The court further noted that under the Freedom of Information Act, such records would be exempt from public disclosure. In a similar case, involving the validity of a NIOSH subpoena for the medical records of several hundred General Motors

---

[17] 42 *Federal Register* 54148 (October 4, 1977).
[18] *E.I. du Pont de Nemours and Co.* vs *Finklea,* 6 OSHC 1167 (D.C.W. Va. 1977).

employees, [19] the court upheld the subpoena, but because there was no compelling need to identify the individuals involved, ordered that medical records be submitted to NIOSH without employee names and addresses.

Thus, the provision in the NIOSH recommendations affording designated medical representatives of the Secretary of Health, Education and Welfare and the Secretary of Labor access to employee medical records, quite common in hazardous substances standards, has been upheld in those cases where it was tested. The NIOSH recommendations also allow the designated medical representative of the employee to review the record. Currently, the Department of Labor is proposing that in addition to providing access to employees' designated physicians, employees themselves should have direct access to their own medical records. Many employer groups vigorously oppose this proposal. [20]

The fifth section of the NIOSH recommendations concerns labeling and posting, and provides that all containers of gaseous and volatile anesthetic agents carry a label stating "Caution: Harmful If Inhaled Continuously." Signs with a similar warning should be posted adjacent to all areas where exposure to anesthetics is likely. Provisions concerning labeling and posting are generally included in OSHA standards governing exposure to toxic substances. In the asbestos lawsuit, employees challenged the wording of the prescribed labels and warnings because, while they stated that exposure to asbestos might be hazardous, they did not mention any particular health hazards. The court upheld the contents of the asbestos label as within the Secretary of Labor's range of discretion. [21] The contents of the NIOSH recommended label would undoubtedly also be within the Secretary's discretion, but it might, nonetheless, be more accurate to qualify the labels so that they carry the statement that inhalation of anesthetics is "potentially" harmful.

The sixth section of the NIOSH criteria states that applicable regulations concerning fire, explosion, and sanitation shall be met when instituting scavenging and engineering controls. The seventh section requires that workers be regularly informed of the possible health effects of exposure to waste anesthetic gases. Many of the OSHA standards go further than the NIOSH recommendations in this regard and require that employers institute formal training programs for all employees exposed to a particular potentially hazardous

---

[19]*General Motors Corporation* vs *Finklea,* 6 OSHC 1976 (W.D. Ohio 1978).
[20]43 *Federal Register* 31371 (July 21, 1978).
[21]*Industrial Union Department* vs. *Hodgson, supra,* note 6.

substance. Such a program would instruct employees in the potential hazards of exposure to the substance, methods of minimizing such exposure, recommended medical surveillance, and the employee's relationship to engineering and work practice controls. The eighth section of the NIOSH criteria sets forth the details of a monitoring program which employers must initiate. Provisions requiring regular monitoring of workplace concentrations of potentially hazardous materials are mentioned in the Act and are included in most OSHA standards pertaining to toxic substances.

The ninth and last section of the NIOSH recommendations concerns maintenance of records. Medical records are to be kept by employers for the duration of an employee's employment plus 20 years. Records of collected air samples are to be kept for at least 20 years and are to be available to exposed employees upon request. This extensive record keeping is justified as necessary and appropriate for the development of information regarding the causes and prevention of occupational hazards related to exposure to a toxic substance. To be useful for this purpose, records must be maintained long enough to allow health effects related to employee exposure to become manifest. Because some health effects do not become manifest for many years, the Department of Labor in promulgating OSHA standards has often required that medical and monitoring records be maintained for extensive periods.[22] The NIOSH recommendations also state that the results of equipment leak tests should be maintained for at least 20 years. The need for this additional record-keeping requirement is somewhat unclear.

The NIOSH section on record keeping should indicate that the results of environmental measurements besides being available to exposed employees will also be available to designated representatives of the Department of Labor and NIOSH. It would also be consistent with recent OSHA standards to require employers to provide employees or their representatives an opportunity to observe the environmental monitoring of employee exposure to toxic substances.

---

[22]Recently, the Department of Labor promulgated a standard requiring employers to retain environmental monitoring records as well as employee medical records, even if the compilation of such records is not required by a specific OSHA standard but is solely done on the employer's initiative. Therefore, hospitals which do maintain records of air samples in their operating rooms and have provided medical examinations to exposed employees are required under OSHA to retain these environmental and medical records. Employers wth fewer than 10 employees are exempted from such record-keeping responsibilities. [43 *Federal Register* 31329 (July 21, 1978)]

In summary, the general approach of the NIOSH recommendations comports with that mandated by the Act and followed in OSHA standards regulating occupational exposure to toxic substances. The wisdom of some of the technical details of the NIOSH recommendations is beyond the scope of this chapter.

An interesting topic which is not mentioned in the NIOSH recommendations on waste anesthetics concerns job assignments of workers who face a particularly great risk of health hazards from occupational exposure. One section of the OSHA standard regulating exposure to asbestos states as follows:

> No employee shall be assigned to tasks requiring the use of respirators if, based upon his most recent examination, an examining physician determines that the employee will be unable to function normally wearing a respirator, or that the safety or health of the employee or other employees will be impaired by his use of a respirator. Such employee shall be rotated to another job or given the opportunity to transfer to a different position whose duties he is able to perform with the same employer, in the same geographical area and with the same seniority, status and rate of pay he had just prior to such transfer, if such a different position is available.[23]

A similar transfer policy might be implemented by an employer with regard to employees occupationally exposed to anesthetics. Candidates for a transfer would most probably be individuals who wished to have children and were concerned about the increased risk of spontaneous abortion and congenital deformities in their offspring, or individuals suffering from liver or kidney conditions which might be aggravated by repeated exposure to anesthetics. The requirement in the asbestos OSHA standard that the transfer be to a position of similar status and pay would be harder to adhere to in a hospital setting. Operating room nurses have a recognized specialty which they would have to relinquish at least temporarily. Similarly, an anesthesiologist would have difficulty in avoiding areas of anesthetic exposure without totally disrupting his or her clinical practice.

In any event, the NIOSH recommendations do not speak to this issue. Nonetheless, employers would be free to initiate transfer policies on their own. Affording employees the right to transfer out of a position involving occupational exposure to a potential health hazard is troublesome when the decision to transfer is made without the consent of the concerned employee, and the transfer is to a position of lesser pay, status, or seniority.

---

[23]29 C.F.R. Section 1910.1001(d)(2)(iv)(c).

Use of OSHA in Private Litigation

OSHA invests the Department of Labor with the authority to cite employers for violations of OSHA's provisions. Attempts by private individuals to sue employers directly in court for OSHA violations have been unsuccessful.[24] The courts have uniformly held that OSHA provides for a governmentally controlled enforcement mechanism and does not create a private right of action that runs in favor of employees.

Despite the fact the a private individual's cause of action cannot be based upon an alleged violation of OSHA, OSHA has had some indirect effects in private litigation. Generally, litigants have attempted to introduce OSHA standards in private lawsuits to prove that a defendant who did not comply with the OSHA requirements was negligent and/or that a product manufactured by a defendant was defective. Attempts to introduce OSHA standards in civil litigation have had disparate results. Some courts have held that proof of failure to comply with OSHA standards constitutes negligence per se,[25] others have said that OSHA standards can provide some evidence of negligence,[26] and a few have held that OSHA standards are inadmissible in civil litigation.[27] The cases in which OSHA has been an issue have all involved the attempt to introduce promulgated OSHA standards into evidence. Evidence of particular OSHA citations or OSHRC adjudications would probably be ruled inadmissible as irrelevant and prejudicial.[28]

Although OSHA places upon employers the primary responsibility for providing a healthful and safe place of employment, the Act will probably have a greater impact on the civil liability of manufacturers of products used in the workplace than on most private employers themselves. This result comes about not through conscious choice but because of the ramifications of workers' compensation laws which foreclose lawsuits by employees against their employers for workplace injuries.[29]

---

[24]*Byrd* vs *Fieldcrest Mills, Inc.,* 496 F.2d 1323 (4th Cir. 1974); *Russel* vs *Bartley,* 494 F.2d 334 (6th Cir. 1974).

[25]*Authur* vs *Flota Mercantile Grain Centra Americana S.A.,* 487 F.2d 561 (5th Cir. 1973).

[26]*Schroeder* vs *C.F. Braun and Co.,* 502 F.2d 235 (7th Cir. 1974).

[27]*Otto* vs *Specialities, Inc.,* 386 F. Supp. 1240 (N. Miss. 1974).

[28]R. Miller, The Occupational Safety and Health Act of 1970 and the Law of Torts, 38 *Law and Contemporary Problems* 612 (1974).

[29]Note, "The Use of OSHA in Products Liability Suits Against the Manufacturers of Industrial Machinery," 11 *Valparaiso University Law Review* 37 (1976).

GENERAL LEGAL PRINCIPLES

As has been discussed, OSHA is directed specifically to issues of workplace safety and health. It is designed to minimize work-related hazards. There are other more general legal principles which traditionally have been utilized by workers once they have become injured on the job.

Individuals suffering occupational diseases can collect workers' compensation benefits from their employer. They may also have a viable lawsuit against third parties based upon negligence or strict liability theories. However, all the remedies potentially available to an injured worker are dependent upon a showing that the occupational exposure in some manner caused the worker's injury or disease. In cases involving individuals occupationally exposed to waste anesthetics, it will be extremely difficult, if not impossible, to prove such a causal relationship. Because individuals occupationally exposed to waste anesthetics will probably, therefore, be unable to benefit from many of these remedies, the remedies will only be described very briefly.

Remedies Against Employers—Workers' Compensation

All states have enacted workers' compensation laws which provide a scheme of employer liability without fault to injured employees based upon insurance concepts. Under workers' compensation, negligence is discarded as the basis of an employer's liability to its employees. To qualify for workers' compensation, an employee must suffer a work-connected injury, i.e., one which arises out of and in the course of employment. It is immaterial whether or not the employer's negligence proximately caused the employee's injury. Occupational diseases, such as silicosis, asbestosis, and lead poisoning, are considered compensable injuries.

The adjudication of disputes concerning an employee's entitlement is made by a special state tribunal, often called a Workers' Compensation Appeals Board. Workers' compensation laws foreclose private lawsuits by an employee against his or her employer. The rule in almost all states is that when workers' compensation laws are applicable, the rights and remedies provided therein are exclusive.[30] An employer is immune from any lawsuit arising out of a work-connected injury suffered by an employee. This immunity extends not only to the claims of the employee but also to claims of the employee's

---

[30] Larson, *Workmen's Compensation* (Desk Ed.) Section 67.00, 1972.

dependents and nondependents which are based on the employee's injuries.[31]

The major advantage of workers' compensation to employees is that because it is a no-fault system, benefits are provided in a wide range of cases. Many workers' compensation laws contain a provision which states that the statute should be construed liberally for the purpose of extending benefits to injured employees. The disadvantage is that the benefit levels tend to be much lower than what an injured employee would recover in court if the employer were found negligent.

In the context of individuals exposed to waste anesthetics, a workers' compensation case could arise, if, for instance, an operating room nurse suffered some sort of liver disease and attempted to receive workers' compensation benefits from the hospital's insurance carrier. Because liver disease is readily contracted in everyday life, the nurse would have difficulty demonstrating that the injury arose out of the hospital environment. As stated before, workers' compensation statutes are construed liberally for the purpose of extending benefits to injured employees. Therefore, for purposes of workers' compensation, a nurse might prevail if he or she could show that employment in the hospital operating room subjected personnel to special risks of liver disease in excess of those experienced by the general public. This "special risk" approach has been allowed in other situations. For example, hospital employees who have contracted infectious disease such as tuberculosis have often been able to recover workers' compensation benefits by proving the special risks of their employment situation.

Remedies against Third Parties

The exclusivity of worker's compensation proceedings applies only to actions by employees against their employers. An employee who sustains an industrial injury, in addition to making a claim for workers' compensation against the employer, is free to bring civil suit for damages against a third party whom the employee claimed caused the injury.

---

[31] In other words, if the spouse of a hospital employee suffered a spontaneous abortion and claimed that this occurred because her husband had been exposed to excessive levels of waste anesthetics, the spouse, as well as the hospital employee, would be unable to maintain a civil action against the employer.

In the hospital context, an injured operating room nurse would not be precluded by workers' compensation laws from bringing an action against an anesthesiologist. Similarly, an injured anesthesiologist would not be precluded from bringing an action against the hospital where he or she practices. The basis of both actions would be that the negligence of the defendant proximately caused the plaintiff's injury. The alleged negligence of a defendant anesthesiologist might consist of work practices which increased the level of waste anesthetics. The alleged negligence of a defendant hospital might consist of non-existent or inadequate environmental monitoring, equipment maintenance, and scavenging devices. If an OSHA standard regulating exposure to waste anesthetics existed, the standard could assist in defining the expected conduct of the hospital and/or anesthesiologist.

Depending on the facts, an injured individual who was occupationally exposed to waste anesthetics might bring an action against the suppliers of the anesthetic gases and the manufacturers of the anesthetic equipment. A special (strict) liability is imposed in the law upon the seller of products. A seller who sells a product in an unreasonably dangerous or defective condition is subject to liability for the harm caused to users of the product even if the seller has exercised all possible care in the preparation and sale of the product.[32] The rationale for this special liability is that public policy demands that the burden of accidental injuries caused by their products be placed upon the companies that market them. Injured workers who were occupationally exposed to asbestos and lead have brought actions against the manufacturers of these products. They maintained that because of the manufacturers' failure to warn of the dangers of chronic exposure, their products were unreasonably dangerous and therefore the manufacturers were subject to strict liability for employees' injuries.[33]

To prevail in any of these third-party lawsuits, an individual plaintiff would need to prove that his or her injury or disease was proximately caused by the defendant's defective product or negligent actions. In the context of occupational disease from chronic exposure to waste anesthetics, this is a substantial legal hurdle. While the disease asbestosis is specifically caused by exposure to asbestos, and lead poisoning is attributable to exposure to lead, the effects of exposure to anesthetic gases are similar to conditions which might occur without exposure. It could be very difficult for a plaintiff to show that chronic

---

[32] *Restatement (Second) of Torts,* Section 402A (1965).
[33] *Borel* vs *Fibreboard Paper Products Corporation,* 493 F.2d 1076 (5th Cir. 1973), *Cert denied* 95 S. Ct. 127 (1974); *Karjala* vs *Johns-Manville Products.* 523 F.2d 155 (8th Cir. 1975).

exposure to certain gases occasioned his or her health problems.[34] Reliance would have to be placed on statistics, but it is unclear how far the courts will allow the use of statistics in attributing disease produced to exposure shown.[35]

CONCLUSIONS

OSHA deals directly with an employer's responsibility to provide its employees a safe and healthful place of employment. As of this date no specific OSHA health and safety standard has been enacted which regulates occupational exposure to waste anesthetics. Nonetheless, employers who make no effort to control and monitor the levels of waste anesthetics might be cited for a violation of OSHA's general duty clause. If the Department of Labor eventually promulgates a standard on waste anesthetics, like all of its standards concerning toxic materials, it will most probably require specific performance levels, environmental monitoring, work practices, medical surveillance, and record keeping.

Because the health effects of occupational exposure to waste anesthetics are similar to those which may occur without exposure, many of the non-OSHA remedies, traditionally utilized by injured workers, will prove unavailing to individuals suffering from health conditions they believe relate to occupational exposure to waste anesthetics.

---

[34]Further complicating the issue is the fact that some of the health effects of anesthetics may take a while to manifest and may result from exposure at more than one source over a period of time.
[35]9 *Am. Jur. Proof of Facts* 719.

EPILOGUE

Twelve years have elapsed since Vaisman's original survey of Russian anesthetists suggesting serious health hazards. Although the intervening years have produced 20 epidemiologic studies conducted in eight countries which largely support her original observation, significant unanswered questions yet remain. A cause-effect relationship between long-term toxicity and anesthetic gas exposure has not been firmly established. Lack of adequate dose-response information makes it difficult to define critical exposure levels or assign risks to various operating room and dental personnel. In addition, few data are available regarding duration and recovery from the associated toxic effects. Future studies must address these critical issues if we are to understand fully the relationship between anesthetic exposure and health.

Nonetheless, significant data continue to accumulate which establish an increased health risk to exposed personnel. The National Institute for Occupational Safety and Health has taken proper lead in recommending precautionary and corrective measures in light of the generally confirming evidence. Few would question our government's motivation in establishing guidelines, but there remain those who contest the seriousness of the issue, cost-effectiveness of its application, and the level of government interference.

While each of us, after carefully reviewing the data, must reserve the right to make our individual decisions, there is an important additional consideration associated with exposure to waste anesthetic gases. Unfortunately, poor work practice on the part of any one individual anesthetist influences not only his own breathing zone, but the escaping gases pollute the breathing zones of others who must work in the same environment. In a sense, we become our brothers' keepers, and the acceptable personal alternative lessens. We as authors remain convinced by the validity of the experimental data, the seriousness of the problem, and the morality of the issue. In good conscience, it is difficult to mount valid arguments against efforts to reduce waste anesthetic gas exposure.